Breastfeeding Special Care Babies

Dedication

This book is dedicated to:

Katy and Marcus, two very special babies, who are now two very special young people

All the many other 'special' babies and their families

All the nursing and medical staff, past and present, of the Exeter Neonatal Unit

And to my Mum, Dad and Mandy

For Baillière Tindall:

Publishing Manager: Inta Ozols
Project Development Manager: Karen Gilmour
Project Manager: Andrea Hill
Designer: Judith Wright

Breastfeeding Special Care Babies

SECOND EDITION

Sandra Lang MPhil RM RGN Dip Ed Cert Ed ENB 405

Foreword by

Dr Felicity Savage FRCP

Honorary Senior Lecturer, Centre for International Child Health,
Institute of Child Health, London

 The Neonatal Nurses Association

BAILLIÈRE TINDALL
EDINBURGH LONDON NEW YORK OXFORD PHILADELPHIA ST LOUIS SYDNEY TORONTO 2002

BAILLIÈRE TINDALL
An imprint of Elsevier Limited

First edition 1997
Second edition 2002
  Reprinted 2003, 2005 (twice)

ISBN 0 7020 2544 5

British Library Cataloguing in Publication Data
A catalogue record for this book is available from the British Library.

Library of Congress Cataloging in Publication Data
A catalog record for this book is available from the Library of Congress.

Note
Medical knowledge is constantly changing. As new information becomes available, changes in treatment, procedures, equipment and the use of drugs become necessary. The author and the publishers have taken care to ensure that the information given in this text is accurate and up to date. However, readers are strongly advised to confirm that the information, especially with regard to drug usage, complies with the latest legislation and standards of practice.

your source for books,
journals and multimedia
in the health sciences
www.elsevierhealth.com

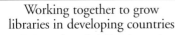

Working together to grow
libraries in developing countries

www.elsevier.com | www.bookaid.org | www.sabre.org

ELSEVIER   BOOK AID International   Sabre Foundation

The
publisher's
policy is to use
**paper manufactured
from sustainable forests**

Printed in China
P/04

Contents

Foreword to the First Edition

Breastfeeding Special Care Babies fills a gap in the literature of breast-feeding. It provides a comprehensive guide for staff in neonatal units and midwives. The book fulfils the promise made in the Introduction, offering a range of conventional and unconventional approaches to feeding the preterm, sick and other vulnerable babies.

Included in the first two chapters are the essential factors which govern a baby's ability to feed and his ability to do so effectively. This leads into the practical aspects of breastfeeding, described clearly and with specific application to the preterm baby. An excellent chapter on expressing breastmilk follows, detailing hand expression, storage and effect of storage and freezing breastmilk. To reduce problems for mothers who express milk over a long period of time, the author describes back massage to stimulate the release of oxytocin and the let-down reflex.

Common breastfeeding problems are dealt with succinctly and include the disadvantages of the all too common use of nipple shields in Chapter 4, and Chapter 5 includes helpful descriptions of relactation. In Chapter 6, milk production is described, and is related to milk expression and the nutritional needs for growth of the low birth weight and sick baby.

For babies with particular feeding problems, for example, babies with cleft palate, Bell's palsy, respiratory and heart problems, alternative methods of feeding are given in great detail with advice on how any difficulties can often be overcome. Midwives will find the sections on physiological jaundice and the use of phototherapy particularly useful, as well as the helpful suggestions on the unsettled baby. An outline of the effect of drugs on breastfeeding refers also to other documents to be consulted for their effects.

Concluding the book are excellent recommendations for the management of breastfeeding on a neonatal or specialist paediatric unit.

Many aspects of breastfeeding wait to be researched, including some of the techniques and skills mentioned. However, common sense always prevails. Tender, loving care and respect of the mother and baby shines through all sections.

I would recommend this book without hesitation.

Dora Henschel, RN, RM, MTD, IBCLC
Co-ordinator of the Joint Breastfeeding Initiative

Foreword to the Second Edition

There is no substitute for practical experience, intelligently and critically gathered, constantly cross-checked against scientific evidence, and reassessed in the light of new knowledge. That is what this book brings to the evolving subject of breastfeeding of special care babies, and practitioners can be confident that it represents the soundest of currently available knowledge about what to do and how to do it. While much attention is now paid to breastfeeding of full term, healthy babies, and the care available for them improves, breastfeeding of babies who are small or sick has remained relatively neglected, and the need to do more for these babies has become urgent.

It is only recently that there has been widespread acceptance of the fact that infants in special care can breastfeed, and that breastmilk is indeed suitable for even the earliest enteral feeds. Many paediatricians and neonatal nurses were trained at a time when breastfeeding and breastmilk were not considered adequate, and scarcely even safe, for the premature or sick infant. It was as if a baby needed to be already strong to withstand such uncertain nurture. Much of our present confidence that a mother's milk is the best, even for a more vulnerable newborn, came from pioneering work in less privileged countries, where greatly improved outcomes followed the use of expressed breastmilk, fed by cup, to low birth weight infants. It has taken much dedicated work to gather the experience needed to convince sceptics that even in western countries very small babies thrive on breastmilk, that it can improve their survival, that they can suckle effectively at a much earlier stage than was formerly believed, and that feeding bottles are usually unnecessary.

However, even when the principles have been established, much work remains for nurses and midwives to acquire the skills to enable mothers to succeed in such a delicate task. Even more work is needed to pass on those skills to others, and the confidence that goes with them, so that effective practices become institutionalised and routine, and so that a high standard of special care is available to all mothers and babies who need it. There are few health professionals who have the necessary skills, and the topic is not yet widely taught. Although the number of infant feeding specialists able to support breastfeeding generally is increasing, there are limited opportunities to specialise and to acquire expertise in the field of special care. Rarer still is Sandra Lang's gift of teaching and sharing practical knowledge in a tactfully authoritative and inspiring way, and her willingness to devote so much time and effort to developing and promoting this subject.

Many schemes for improved neonatal care which include increasing the use of expressed breastmilk, or feeding directly from the breast at an earlier stage, founder simply because of poor technique. This book contains detailed user-friendly descriptions of techniques known to be effective, and is thus an essential aid for improvement – surpassed only by the author teaching the techniques in person. The ability to attach a premature baby to the breast, to cup feed one who cannot yet suckle enough, and knowledge of how to assess an infant's capability, and to strike the optimum balance between different methods, are also vital for implementation of the most well intentioned policies.

A gift for sharing practical knowledge, as well as care and concern for mothers and babies, is apparent throughout this book. The first edition has been read and used all over the world, reflecting the author's extensive international experience, and her understanding of the common needs of mothers, babies and health professionals everywhere. The second edition is up to date in the light of new research findings, experience of implementing the Baby Friendly Initiative, and training of health care professionals in a number of different countries in Europe and elsewhere.

Good practice for special care babies has much in common with good practice for other babies, and the basis for both is the same. Therefore, much of the information contained in these pages is also of value for the non-specialist, in helping the mother of any infant to breastfeed. This book can be confidently recommended to all who are concerned with the protection, promotion and support of breastfeeding, with advancing the Baby Friendly Initiative, and with the better care of newborns, detailing as it does the practical wisdom which both policy and science need to move ahead.

Dr Felicity Savage

Acknowledgements

I would like to thank the following people who have shared with me their professional expertise, wisdom and warmth in helping mothers and babies to breastfeed – they have contributed a great deal to this book. They are: Nola Gendle, Mary-Anne Shields, Marlene Harris, Pamela Bell, Tracy Cann, Sharon Hore, Dr Marie Hanlon, Helen Shoesmith and all the midwifery, nursing and medical staff at the Exeter Neonatal Unit; the breastfeeding counsellors from the Exeter branch of the National Childbirth Trust; Dora Henschel; the Royal College of Midwives Breastfeeding Working Group, particularly Chloe Fisher and Sally Inch, for their helpful suggestions and advice; and the Neonatal Nurses Association.

I owe special thanks to Gabriella Palmer for her wonderful way with words and her generosity in helping me to express clearly some of the more complex parts of the text.

I am also grateful to Fiona Dykes and Kate Dinwoodie of the Department of Midwifery Studies at the University of Central Lancashire; Liz Jones of the North Staffs Neonatal Unit for some of the photographs used in this book; and to Daphne Paley-Smith for her lovely line drawings.

My thanks also go to my friends and family for their support and encouragement, and to my colleagues in the Department of Midwifery Studies at the University of Central Lancashire – who probably know this book by heart!

I have left two very special acknowledgements until last. Early in the 1970s, I travelled to a town called Janakpur in southern Nepal as a teacher with Voluntary Service Overseas. It was here and in the surrounding villages that I spent many hours behind mud walls with the women and children in their compounds. I observed and learned about the subtle art of breastfeeding, and saw the alternative methods that were used to feed babies born either prematurely or very small, and who were unable to breastfeed exclusively at birth. Many of these babies survived because of the skill of their mothers in using cups and rudimentary breastfeeding supplementers. All of them eventually succeeded in breastfeeding. I do not know or remember the names of many of these women or of their babies who taught me so much, but I am deeply grateful for the education I received from them.

And finally, I am indebted to the many mothers, fathers and babies whose experiences of breastfeeding have made this book possible.

Second edition

The completion of this second edition is almost entirely due to Suzanne Hearnshaw and her daughter, Anna, who required special care for several months and for whom breastfeeding has been so much more than simply nutrition.

I owe many thanks to Jane Putsey of the Breastfeeding Network for helping me at such short notice, to Joan Joyner who provided the commas, to Allison Watts of the National Childbirth Trust for her very constructive and thoughtful comments, and to Olivia Lowendahl for reading it all! I am particularly grateful to Jenny Watts and her daughter, Abigail, who once again showed me how wonderfully clever new babies are.

Since the first edition was published I have again had the privilege of seeing mothers breastfeeding their babies in a number of different lands far from mine. On each occasion I have been struck by how much there is still to learn about breastfeeding and how ingenious mothers, health professionals and babies are in the face of adversity. I continue to be indebted to the mothers and fathers and babies whose lives I have glimpsed and who unknowingly have once again contributed to this book.

Sandra Lang

Katy – A Special Baby

The baby on the front cover is Katy Taylor. She and her parents have contributed more to this book than they will ever realize, and I am grateful to her parents for giving permission to use her photograph.

Katy was born at 24 weeks' gestation on 23 March 1990, weighing 756 grams. She was ventilated for a total of 48 days from birth and required oxygen via a headbox for a further 15 days, before having oxygen via nasal cannulae. This was eventually discontinued one month after discharge. She was in the neonatal intensive care unit for a total of 74 days, before being transferred to the special care unit for low-dependency care.

She was initially fed intravenously. She began to have expressed breastmilk on day 4 via a nasal gastric tube at 0.5 mL per hour. Thereafter she received:

- continuous pump feeds for 51 days from day 4 to day 54
- 1-hourly bolus feeds for 9 days from day 55 to day 63
- 2-hourly bolus feeds for 8 days from day 64 to day 71
- 3-hourly bolus feeds for 11 days from day 72 to day 82
- 3–4-hourly bolus feeds (as required) for 27 days from day 83 to day 104 and was breastfeeding on demand from day 105.

Her breastfeeding history

On day 48 she had her first 'lick' at the breast (this was also the day on which she was extubated). She was approximately 31 weeks old.

On day 49 she had a few gentle sucks at the breast.

On day 52 she had a short breastfeed (requiring supplementing afterwards by gastric tube).

On day 59 she had two slightly longer breastfeeds (requiring supplementing afterwards by gastric tube).

Between days 60 and 102 she was having at least one to four breastfeeds a day. The nasal tube was gradually removed with occasional oral tube feeds given.

On day 74 she had her first cup feed. Altogether, she had 38 cup feeds during the next 29 days. Amounts taken were between 5 mL and 85 mL. The majority of the cup feeds were in excess of her fluid requirement as charted.

On day 103 she no longer required any tube feeds or cup feeds, for she was then totally breastfed.

By day 105 she was demand feeding approximately every 2–4 hours. She was discharged weighing 2532 grams, on day 115.

Katy stopped breastfeeding completely when she was three and a half years old. She is now at school, and is considered to be very bright. She goes horse-riding, cycling and loves her ballet class. She is tall for her age and has been remarkably healthy, having been hospitalized only once since she was discharged from the neonatal unit.

And now, in this second edition, let Katy speak for herself:

… My name is Katy Lauren Taylor and I live on Dartmoor. I am 11 years old. I live with my mum and go to the local primary school. My best friends are Anna and Andrew. I have three cats, Breachin, Pushkin and Clover, and a rabbit called Pixie. I also have two horses and am horse crazy! One of my horses is loaned from a local trekking centre and the other one is a pony, called Dan Y Lan Jolly Roger or Dunny for short! I take modern dance lessons every Thursday. I have done three grades in ballet. I am also in the school band and am in grade one for clarinet.

Introduction

This is a book about the challenges of breastfeeding. It is a practical guide, which has grown out of the many and varied experiences of mothers and fathers, whose babies were admitted to a neonatal unit; the health professionals, who with patience, imagination and skill helped many of the babies to begin life nourished with their mother's own breastmilk, and go home successfully breastfeeding; lay breastfeeding counsellors and health professionals, who provided continuing support to the families for a long time after the babies had gone home; and the mothers, fathers, their babies, and health professionals in countries far from mine, whose fresh and innovative approaches to breastfeeding challenges were inspirational.

Many of the practices considered in the following chapters are fundamental to successful breastfeeding: for example, correct positioning and attachment. Many are supported by good scientific evidence; others have grown out of practical experience in a neonatal, transitional care or paediatric unit, where breastfeeding may not be straightforward. Some of these practices have proved beneficial in helping both the mother and baby to establish breastfeeding – they are, therefore, included in this book. These practices include using the breastfeeding supplementer, the cup, and back massage. As a result, this book offers a range of conventional and unconventional approaches to the many challenging situations that can arise in hospital units caring for preterm, sick and other vulnerable babies – indeed, in any situation where breastfeeding takes place. It is aimed at protecting the unique role of the mother who, having made the commitment to breastfeed, has a right to succeed, wherever she lives in the world.

Throughout this book the mother is referred to as 'she' and the baby as 'he'. This is to ensure there is no confusion in reading the text.

Sandra Lang MPhil, RM, RGN, Dip Ed, Cert Ed, ENB 405, is co-director of the 'Breastfeeding: Practice and Policy Course' held annually at the Centre for International Child Health at the Institute of

Child Health in London. She is an independent breastfeeding advisor and teacher. Her interest in the ways preterm or sick infants are fed began over 25 years ago while she was working in southern Nepal, and her work since then has been highly acclaimed both nationally and internationally.

1

The basics of breastfeeding

1.1 THE CHALLENGE OF BREASTFEEDING

There is no doubt that breastfeeding is by far the best way to feed a term, healthy baby. But what about a baby who needs admission to a neonatal or paediatric unit? There is a wealth of evidence emerging that breastmilk and breastfeeding are as important for the vulnerable baby as for the healthy baby.[1] Breastmilk helps to protect babies in so many different ways that it seems illogical not to use this remarkable fluid as a vital part of their medication and treatment. Consider what breastmilk contains: factors that protect a baby against infection, factors that aid growth and neurological development, factors reducing susceptibility to certain diseases in childhood and even into adulthood – and there are health benefits for the mother as well. Breastmilk is therefore as important to the long-term wellbeing of a vulnerable baby, as ventilation is to the baby's short-term survival.

How can we help the mother to breastfeed when her baby is preterm, ill or in need of special care? The mother's success or otherwise often depends upon the environment in which she finds herself, and the attitudes of those who care for her. Where breastfeeding and breastmilk are viewed positively and considered beneficial for the baby, and the staff are well trained in the skills needed by the mother, she is likely to succeed. In an environment where the long-term value of breastfeeding is not thought important, her chances are greatly reduced.

It is possible to have an academic, detached understanding of breastmilk and breastfeeding in general, particularly in an era of evidence-based medicine, and there is certainly no shortage of scientific evidence about the benefits of breastfeeding and breastmilk. However, simply saying that a baby needing special care should breastfeed (or receive his mother's breastmilk) is not enough. Anyone working with a mother who wants to breastfeed and whose baby requires special care will know that the practical side of breastfeeding must be equally well understood. If we are responsible for helping a mother to breastfeed, we must have at our fingertips:

◆ the skills to help her initiate and sustain lactation (the process of producing breastmilk)
◆ the skill to support her for many days or weeks – or even months – until the baby is able to breastfeed
◆ the skill to decide which of the different methods of feeding will help a baby in special care to establish breastfeeding
◆ the skills to help the mother maintain healthy breasts or cope with any breast problems that might occur.

It is these skills that empower a mother to nurture her baby. Without them, we cannot give mother or child the help they both need to succeed in breastfeeding against all the odds.

For many mothers there is an overwhelming physiological and psychological need to 'help' their baby, particularly after the birth. Mothers cannot always put into words how they feel, but very often giving their own breastmilk satisfies part of this overwhelming need – even when a baby is not likely to live for very long. We should always ask a mother if she wants to express her breastmilk for her baby – it is her right to nourish her own child, and with our help this is usually achievable.

When a mother has made a commitment to breastfeed or express her milk, it is essential that she can be fully supported by knowledgeable and skilled health professionals who appreciate her unique role in providing not only a source of nourishment for her baby, but an important component of the baby's medical and emotional treatment as well.

The mother is often as emotionally vulnerable as her baby is clinically vulnerable. She needs constant reassurance that her breastmilk is special, and that she is the only person who is able to:

◆ soothe her baby by holding him next to her breast with its own special comforting scent and the sound of her heartbeat
◆ continue the symbiotic non-verbal relationship started in the womb and which through breastfeeding contributes to a close and loving relationship
◆ provide her baby with a unique 'tailor-made' food, containing her own specific antibodies and other protective properties.

No health professional can ever provide this very intimate care. A mother needs to know that her milk and her ability to breastfeed are a vital part of her baby's treatment, for then she may feel she is an important part of the team of people caring for him. Many parents can feel their baby is not really theirs until they take him home. To avoid this there must be a partnership in which parents and health professionals respect and value each other's role and skills.

The reality of having a baby admitted to a neonatal or paediatric unit, for whatever reason, is a stressful and frequently frightening experience. Parents are often confused by the technology and environment, they may feel helpless,[2] guilty, afraid, anxious about their baby's survival or long-term outcome. Complications during the pregnancy or labour may leave the mother unwell, and she may have seen her baby for only a short time after delivery before he was whisked away to a neonatal unit. Even when the reason for admission is not life-threatening or potentially serious, the mother can feel emotionally drained, insecure and lacking confidence in her ability to care for her new baby. Over time parents do become familiar with a specialist unit – but it is from that very first day that the environment has to be sympathetic to the mother who wishes to breastfeed, and that can be the real challenge.

Many mothers do not succeed in breastfeeding on a neonatal unit. Some cite the lack of support from medical and nursing staff as part of the reason, some cite the conflicting advice they are given, and some the lack of practical help they receive. To help mothers to succeed in breastfeeding, the information contained in the rest of this chapter and in the following chapters is aimed at supporting them to overcome any challenges that may occur during a baby's stay in a neonatal, transitional care or paediatric unit or even in the postnatal ward, and when the baby goes home. By giving a mother who wishes to establish breastfeeding the confidence and the skills to succeed, regardless of the gestation or condition of her baby at birth, we also give her and her family a positive experience which they will remember for the rest of their lives.

1.2 THE BENEFITS OF BREASTMILK AND OF BREASTFEEDING

Breastmilk is much more than simply nutrition – it is a unique and complex fluid containing well over a hundred documented constituents. Many scientific papers examining its biochemical properties have been written and so many new discoveries about its properties are constantly being made that it is difficult to keep up with them all. Breastmilk is considered to be a 'living' fluid,[3] for in addition to its nutrient content it contains antibacterial, antiviral, anti-infective and antiparasitic factors, as well as hormones, enzymes, specialized growth factors and immunological properties.[4]

The benefits of breastmilk and of breastfeeding are many. On a global level it significantly reduces infant and childhood morbidity and mortality,[5] and probably contributes far more to the health and wellbeing of a nation than perhaps is realized or acknowledged. It is shocking to realize that, according to the World Health Organization, 'as many as

10% of all deaths of children under five could be prevented by a modest increase in the breastfeeding rate worldwide'.[6] Consider the following global statistics.

Babies who do not breastfeed:

◆ are at least two and a half times more likely to suffer an episode of illness
◆ in their first year of life are up to three times more likely to die of respiratory infection compared with babies who are exclusively breastfed.

Babies who do not exclusively breastfeed:

◆ are up to 25 times more likely to die from diarrhoea in the first 6 months of life.

Babies who receive formula milk:

◆ particularly if they are preterm, are 6–10 times more likely to develop the potentially fatal gut condition known as necrotizing enterocolitis, if given only formula milk and not given breastmilk as the first enteral feed
◆ are twice as likely to suffer from acute otitis media compared with babies who are exclusively breastfed.

Note: **Exclusive** breastfeeding is when the baby receives all his nutrition **at** his mother's breast; **breastmilk feeding** is when a baby receives milk which is **expressed** from his mother and is given by gastric tube, cup, breastfeeding supplementer or bottle.

Many babies require expensive treatment in hospital if they are not breastfed or do not receive breastmilk. The financial burden upon a health service is huge. According to the UK Department of Health:

> *It is estimated that the NHS spends £35 million per year in England and Wales in treating gastroenteritis in bottle-fed infants and that for each 1% increase in breastfeeding at 13 weeks, a saving of £500 000.00 in the treatment of gastroenteritis would be achieved.*[7]

1.2.1 Benefits of breastmilk to the baby

Research on breastmilk indicates that a baby receives a number of important short-term and long-term benefits because of the factors it contains. Many of these benefits appear to continue into childhood and beyond. For example, a study in England found that 66 preterm babies who had received donor breastmilk alone or in addition to their mothers' milk, had lower blood pressures at age 13–16 years, compared with 64 preterm babies given preterm formula milks.[8] A study in Western Australia followed up a large group of children from birth to 6 years and found a significantly lower prevalence of childhood asthma at 6 years in the children who had been breastfed for at least 4 months.[9] Similarly, in Scotland a group of children were followed up from birth to 7 years. The children were found to have a significantly reduced incidence of respiratory illness if they had been exclusively breastfed for at least 15 weeks, compared with children who had been formula-fed or partially breastfed.[10]

Other benefits include:

◆ a reduced incidence of gastrointestinal and respiratory infections during the neonatal period[11,12]
◆ increased protection against dental caries[13,14]
◆ a lower incidence of otitis media[15,16]
◆ a lower incidence of juvenile onset diabetes[17,18]
◆ a reduced mortality rate among preterm and low-birthweight babies from necrotizing enterocolitis[19]
◆ a possible reduction in the incidence of some childhood cancers (lymphoma and Hodgkin's disease)[20]
◆ a reduction in the severity of certain allergic conditions[21]
◆ the presence of specific growth factors in breastmilk which are important in the development and maturation of the brain, retina and central nervous system.[22,23]

1.2.2 Benefits of the mechanical action of breastfeeding to the baby

It is not only the breastmilk itself that is beneficial to a baby but also the mechanical action of breastfeeding. A baby has to open his mouth widely with his tongue down and out over his bottom gum in order to breastfeed effectively. The tongue then remains in that position while wave-like peristaltic movements take place throughout the tongue, from the tip to the back. With the mother's breast tissue far into the baby's mouth, the milk is removed by the wave-like action squeezing the breast tissue against the hard palate and pushing the milk out of the milk reservoirs (lactiferous sinuses – Fig. 1.1) into the throat, where it is swallowed. The action involved in the baby suckling (taking milk from the breast) from the mother's breast is thought to optimally exercise the muscles in the soft palate. Muscles such as the tensor muscle of the soft palate (tensor palati), for example, are optimally enhanced, which helps keep the eustachian tubes open, thus reducing the incidence of 'glue ear' or otitis media with a discharge when the child is older.[16] Babies most at risk of this condition are those born prematurely or with cleft abnormalities,[24] or babies with Down's syndrome.

There is some evidence to suggest that babies who breastfeed have fewer problems with the spacing and evenness of their teeth.[14] It is

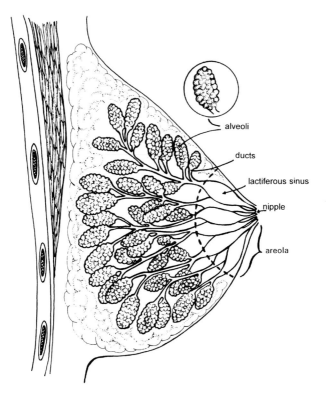

alveoli

ducts

lactiferous sinus

nipple

areola

Figure 1.1 Anatomy of the breast (reproduced with permission from UNICEF).

suggested that this is because the mechanical action of breastfeeding leads to a well-shaped jaw. Some researchers claim that breastfeeding also leads to clearer speech in later childhood.[25]

1.2.3 Benefits to the mother

There is increasing evidence of long-term health benefits from breast-feeding for the mother too. These include:

◆ a reduction in the incidence of premenopausal breast cancer and some types of ovarian cancer[26–28]
◆ a lower incidence of long bone and hip fractures in women over the age of 65;[29] no increased risk of osteoporosis[30]
◆ a delay in the return of fertility[31,32]
◆ helping the mother to lose weight naturally – though for some mothers weight loss may not occur until after the baby has stopped breastfeeding,[33] and for others it may not happen at all, or the

mother notices that her weight distribution is simply different from her pre-pregnancy days!

Some of these benefits may be intensified by the number of times a mother breastfeeds with successive children and the length of each lactation. The effect on breast cancer is an example.[26]

In the first few days after birth, the increased release of the hormone oxytocin helps the uterus to return to its normal size more quickly, reducing the risk of serious haemorrhage in the postnatal period. Some mothers may experience the process of uterine involution as lower abdominal pain (after-pains) and/or increased loss of blood during feeding or milk expression. These events are both normal (with after-pains being more common in mothers breastfeeding after a second pregnancy than after a first pregnancy).

The psychological benefits to the relationship between the mother and her baby are of paramount importance. Breastfeeding is not simply a form of nutrition, it is part of the nurturing process, fundamental to the overall long-term wellbeing of the whole family group – and as such has benefits for all of society.

1.2.4 The practical benefits of breastfeeding

Breastmilk is free! There is no need for a mother to spend extra money on a special diet because she is breastfeeding. Certainly she has to eat adequate, well-balanced meals, but she should do this whether or not she is breastfeeding. Little equipment has to be bought for successful breastfeeding, so more money is available for other necessities. Other advantages are:

- ◆ Breastfeeding produces few by-products, therefore there is little waste – and the baby's stools are sweet-smelling.
- ◆ Breastmilk is always at the correct temperature.
- ◆ It is constantly available and requires no preparation.
- ◆ It is portable, making travel easier as little equipment is needed.
- ◆ It is easy to feed at night.
- ◆ For the term baby, the milk is nutritionally perfect.
- ◆ It is 'environmentally friendly' – there is no processing involved, no packaging and nothing to throw away.

1.3 ANATOMY AND PHYSIOLOGY OF THE LACTATING BREAST

The breasts are remarkable glands. They are capable of producing sufficient milk to totally sustain a baby's nutritional needs for the first

6 months of life,[34] and are capable of making a valuable contribution to the baby's diet for at least the next 2 years.[35]

Each breast contains 15–25 lobes of glandular tissue. Each lobe is further divided into smaller lobes, which contain thousands of alveoli. These are clusters of tiny sacs lined with milk-producing cells, known as the acini cells. The sacs are surrounded by a network of capillary blood vessels from which the individual constituents are taken to synthesize breastmilk under the influence of the hormone prolactin. The sacs are also surrounded by muscle (myoepithelial) cells arranged in a basket-like weave. The hormone oxytocin makes these muscles contract, squeezing the milk into the small ductal tubes of the alveoli, and then into the larger ductal tubes. These eventually drain into the 10–15 distensible ducts which store the milk within the area of the areola, known as lactiferous sinuses (see Fig. 1.1). When a baby suckles, he compresses these sinuses between his tongue and hard palate, by means of a wave-like movement of his tongue. The milk is forced into the 10–15 small, narrow tubes, which lead out to the surface of the nipple, and is then ejected into the baby's mouth.

The tip of the nipple is very sensitive indeed. This is because there are many nerve endings present in this small area. These nerve endings are unmyelinated, which means they are extremely sensitive, and when the nipple is damaged the pain is exquisitely intense.

Not all the lobes of the breast are productive during the complete lactation period, or necessarily for each individual lactation.[36]

The shape and size of breasts differ greatly, but only rarely does this affect their primary function of providing a baby with nourishment.

1.3.1 The initiation of lactation

Lactation is possible as early as 16 weeks after conception, even if a pregnancy ends at this time for any reason.[37] It is the inhibitory effects of the placental hormones, particularly progesterone, that usually delay milk production until birth and the delivery of the placenta. Indeed, any fragments of placental material left in the uterus after delivery can delay the onset of lactation, until they are naturally or surgically removed.[37] Once the blood levels of progesterone have fallen, which usually occurs after 2–3 days, the composition of the milk significantly changes and the volume rapidly increases. The continuing production of milk is thereafter dependent on the regular removal of a quantity of milk and subsequent refilling of the breasts.

Initially it is the maintenance of optimal hormonal levels that is necessary for the establishment of lactation. The most important of these hormones are prolactin, which stimulates the initial alveolar production of milk, and oxytocin, which controls the milk 'let-down' reflex or milk flow by causing the myoepithelial cells to contract. This hormonal control is particularly important during the first few weeks of lactation when the quantity of breastmilk required to sustain the baby is being established. Around 6 weeks after the initiation of lactation it is the efficient drainage of the breast at regular intervals which becomes the main factor in the production of breastmilk rather than the influence of prolactin. It is then that the feedback inhibitor of lactation (see below), which locally controls milk production in the breast, becomes important.

1.3.2 Three important hormones

For many mothers of healthy, term babies the process of breastfeeding is initiated and sustained with the minimum of problems. For these mothers, understanding the way the hormones of lactation work is interesting but rarely of critical importance. However, for the mothers of preterm and otherwise vulnerable babies, knowledge of the hormonal influences on lactation can really help to make breastfeeding more likely to succeed.

Prolactin

The hormone prolactin works by direct nipple stimulation. When the baby suckles, sensory impulses pass from the nipple area to the anterior part of the pituitary gland in the brain. This is where prolactin is produced and secreted into the blood. When the prolactin in the blood comes into contact with the acini cells, milk is produced. The level of prolactin in the blood remains high for up to 75–90 minutes after a feed; thus suckling at one feed helps stimulate production of the milk for the next.[38] Prolactin levels are higher at night than during the day, though why this should be so is a mystery.

Oxytocin

The hormone oxytocin can be stimulated both before and during breastfeeding. Again, stimulation of the nipple is important. Sensory impulses pass from the breast to the posterior part of the pituitary gland and oxytocin is released into the blood. The milk flows in response to oxytocin making the myoepithelial cells in the alveoli contract. This happens as the baby suckles.

However, oxytocin is also stimulated by other sensory pathways. The mother's milk may begin to flow in response to her seeing her baby, hearing him, touching him, smelling him, thinking about him, and in anticipating breastfeeding. This is known as the 'let-down' reflex. However, if the mother is in pain, if she is worried, or if she is distressed for any reason, her oxytocin response may be delayed or work less efficiently, causing her milk to flow more slowly or to temporarily stop flowing. It is easy to see why this often happens to a mother with a baby in a neonatal unit.

Feedback inhibitor of lactation

In recent years a protein has been identified which is secreted within the breast itself. This protein, known as the feedback inhibitor of lactation (FIL), causes the production of milk to be reduced or even to stop.[39] As the quantity of milk builds up in the breast the amount of FIL also increases, gradually slowing the rate of milk production. As milk is removed, by suckling or expression, the level of FIL falls and the speed of milk production rises again. This protein helps protect the breast from the effects of becoming too full. It may also be why some mothers feel that one of their breasts works more efficiently than the other. It also explains why when a baby does not breastfeed regularly or effectively, milk production gradually diminishes, as the breast gets the 'message' that less milk is required.

1.3.3 Artificial stimulation of lactation

Mothers of babies admitted to a neonatal or paediatric unit may not be able to initiate or maintain lactation by breastfeeding. They may have to wait a few days or weeks before breastfeeding is possible. Therefore they may be reliant on artificial methods for stimulating milk production and expressing their breastmilk. These include massage techniques, the mechanical breast pump, the hand breast pump, or hand-expression. Whichever method is chosen, the normal stimuli of breastfeeding are absent. This can have an effect on the mother's long-term chances of maintaining her milk supply and of establishing exclusive breastfeeding.

The mother's let-down reflex responds to a number of different stimuli, which as already mentioned include touching, seeing and hearing her baby, as well as her baby's own particular scent. These stimuli may be partially or totally missing when artificial expression is necessary. In addition, situations that may condition a response before a baby feeds, such as thinking about the baby or physical closeness, may be similarly affected if a mother has to express in a setting far from her baby. Temporary inhibition of her let-down response may occur when a mother is subjected to sudden and unpleasant physical or physiological stimuli, such as may be experienced on a neonatal or paediatric unit. This applies particularly when a mother is under acute stress, although minor or chronic stress does not appear to permanently affect the milk supply in the long term.[37] Nevertheless, short-term variations in milk production can psychologically affect the mother's confidence, and if this is compounded by insufficient support from health professionals or family members, the mother may indeed find it difficult to sustain her milk production for any prolonged period. Ways of overcoming these difficulties are described in the next two chapters.

1.4 THE VARIABILITY, VOLUME AND SEQUENCE OF MILK PRODUCTION

Breastmilk is a constantly changing fluid, varying in composition, and sweet to taste. It varies:

◆ during an individual feed (i.e. fore-milk through to hind-milk)
◆ throughout the course of the day[40]
◆ with the stage of lactation
◆ between different mothers
◆ in the same mother between the two breasts and in different pregnancies[41]
◆ between preterm and term milk,[42] most noticeable in the first 4 to 6 weeks after delivery
◆ with maternal diet, which may also influence its composition[43,44]
◆ with exercise, which may increase the lactose content of the milk.[45]

1.4.1 How much breastmilk is produced?

It takes approximately 6 weeks for a mother to establish her milk supply. During this time she will notice that her supply increases dramatically in the first 5–6 days after delivery. In the first 2–3 days colostrum is produced in relatively small quantities of between 1 mL and 10 mL at each breastfeed or expression (though it may be more). Mothers feeding a second or third baby may produce more milk or colostrum than when they previously breastfed; this may be because the prolactin receptors in the breast have already been primed. Thereafter the quantity of milk produced rises dramatically from approximately 50–70 mL at each feed or expression on day 4 or 5, to 80–120 mL by day 6 or 7. By approximately 6 weeks most mothers have established an average milk output of around 750–800 mL per day.[46] Mothers who produce milk with a low energy content may produce larger volumes than this, as their babies suckle more to satisfy their needs.[47] From around 6 weeks if milk is removed from the breast, the same quantity is produced to replace it. The more efficiently the milk is removed, the more is produced. Also, increasing the number of times that a mother breastfeeds or expresses milk enables her to produce more milk over a 24-hour period. Conversely, if a baby receives formula supplements or a dummy, milk production may be reduced proportionately.

The majority of mothers produce enough breastmilk for their babies for at least the first 6 months. The volume of milk they produce remains relatively constant, and the constituents in the milk change to meet the baby's changing nutritional needs.[48] The quantity of milk naturally decreases once complementary foods are introduced at around 6 months. This is when breastmilk is no longer sufficient on its own, though breastfeeding still remains a valuable part of the baby's diet and wellbeing.

1.4.2 The colour and appearance of breastmilk at different stages of milk production

The colour of human milk is not indicative of its nutritional state. Initially, colostrum is produced: this is a thick, viscous fluid which can be creamy in appearance or look more like plasma. Over the following 2–3 weeks the milk appears less dense and more watery as the colostrum is diluted by the increasing milk volume. It changes gradually from a creamy-white appearance to a blueish-white colour. When the mother and her baby decide to reduce breastfeeding and the frequency of feeding begins to lessen, the milk becomes whiter or more creamy in appearance, and may once again resemble colostrum.

Throughout an individual feed or expression the colour of the milk may also vary slightly. Milk produced at the beginning of a feed appears more watery than the milk produced towards the end, which appears more creamy. These are the two extremes which are commonly known as 'fore-milk' and 'hind-milk'. However, there is no sudden change from fore-milk to hind-milk, they are part of a continuum. Fore-milk has a high water content and contains much of the protein and lactose. As the feed or expression continues the level of fat gradually increases while the protein and lactose levels fall. The energy the baby needs is mostly in the fat-rich part of the milk, which is why it is important for a baby to finish a feed on each breast himself and for the feed not to be 'timed' by either the mother or carer. The fat-rich milk is the hind-milk.

1.5 THE COMPOSITION OF BREASTMILK

There are three identifiable stages of lactation: production of colostrum, transitional milk and mature milk (Fig. 1.2).

1.5.1 Colostrum

Colostrum has an almost medicinal quality, making it an extremely valuable substance for any baby, and essential for preterm and ill babies.

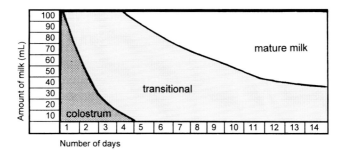

Figure 1.2 The sequence of milk production.

Its functions are still not completely understood,[49] although protection from infection is certainly one of its major roles. It is secreted in the first 3–4 days following birth. Thereafter, it gradually changes into mature milk over a period of 10–15 days, during which time the milk increases in volume, and continues to change subtly in composition. Colostrum is produced in smaller quantities than mature milk – from as little as 1–10 mL at each feed or expression – but the range is considerable (5–100 mL).[50] Despite the small quantity produced, colostrum provides sufficient fluid and nutrients in the first few days of life for a term, healthy baby.

Colostrum is especially rich in proteins, particularly the immunoglobulins IgM, IgG and secretory IgA, and also lactoferrin and lysozymes, which together with the macrophages, lymphocytes and neutrophils (active cells) protect the newborn infant from infections – especially those to which the mother has previously been exposed and has become immune. Secretory IgA is a particularly important immunoglobulin, as it is thought to line the surface of the intestine, thereby protecting a baby from gastrointestinal infections. Another important protein in colostrum, present in concentrations five times greater than in mature milk, is epidermal growth factor (EGF).[51] This is known to stimulate cellular growth in a number of areas of the body.[52] In the intestines EGF leads to an increase in the size of the villi, and helps seal the mucosa so that large molecules cannot penetrate the gut wall into the blood circulation. This is thought to help protect the baby from food allergies, intolerances and sensitivities. **The concentration of growth factors is even higher in the colostrum and in the milk of a mother giving birth to a preterm baby.** This is important information for mothers, for these growth factors help to mature the gut wall soon after delivery and thus protect the baby from potentially life-threatening pathogens.

Apart from its anti-infective role, colostrum has a mild but nevertheless important laxative effect. This helps to clear meconium from the body and thereby prevent the reabsorption of bilirubin, which may cause or increase the severity of jaundice in the early days of life.[53]

In some cultures it is common not to give colostrum to new babies. However, several studies have suggested that it is valuable not only in preventing disease in vulnerable preterm babies, but also in treating infections.[54,55] Indeed, there is evidence of its therapeutic use in ayurvedic medicine (in the Indian subcontinent) to treat certain skin and eye infections in the general population.[56] In Japan, an antibiotic (lactofelicine) has been developed from human colostral proteins. This substance is claimed to be strong enough to kill the bacteria that cause food poisoning within 1 hour. Beneficial gut bacteria are left unharmed by the substance, which is active against *Escherichia coli, Listeria* and other bacteria causing diarrhoea.[54] Colostrum has, therefore, a vitally important role in the initial protection and wellbeing of all babies, particularly those requiring special care.

1.5.2 Mature human milk

The major constituents of breastmilk are fat, protein, carbohydrate, water, vitamins, minerals and trace elements, as well as hormones, enzymes, growth factors, immunological properties and protective factors.

Fat

Fat is essential for normal human development. According to one writer,[57] it forms an integral component of all cellular membranes, transports fat-soluble vitamins and hormones, and provides fatty acids which are crucial for brain development. It is also the principal source of energy in human milk, providing between 40% and 60% of the baby's total energy intake.[58] The fats of human milk are easily digested and absorbed by a baby, with up to 85–95% being utilized in the term baby, falling to approximately 65–80% or less in extremely preterm babies.[59,60]

Triglycerides (triacylglycerols) are the main constituents of milk fat (98–99%).[57] These are readily broken down into free fatty acids and monoglycerides by lipases and bile salts. These lipases are present in the lingual and gastric secretions of term and preterm babies. One of the products of the breakdown of milk fats is monolauryl, a substance with antibacterial, antiviral and antifungal properties,[57] which may contribute to the activation of the baby's defence mechanism even before the gastric phase of digestion.

Human breastmilk itself contains two further lipases: bile salt stimulated lipase and lipoprotein lipase. Bile salt stimulated lipase (BSSL) is activated in the baby's small intestine,[61] where it further contributes to the digestion of fat, compensating for the low levels of pancreatic lipase and bile salt activity in newborn babies. It possibly also improves fat absorption when a mixture of formula and the mother's own milk is given to the baby.[57] The function of lipoprotein lipase (LPL) in milk or in the baby is not fully understood, although it is thought to contribute to the breakdown of the triglycerides into free fatty acids and monoglycerides during storage,[61,62] and is active even at 4 °C.[48]

The free fatty acids in the milk have been shown to be the most important source of energy for the baby; the lipases in milk make them available even before the intestinal phase, thereby improving the energy supply. This helps to make the fat in breastmilk more easily absorbed. Pasteurization of human milk significantly reduces this absorption, possibly because the milk lipases are destroyed.[63] Breastmilk is also particularly rich in long-chain fatty acids, which have an important role in brain development and the myelinization of the nerves.[64] Approximately one-quarter of the brain is composed of these fatty acids, of which arachidonic acid (AA) and docosahexaenoic acid (DHA) are the major components. As with many human milk factors, DHA is more concentrated in colostrum,[65] and the milk of mothers of preterm babies contains more DHA and AA than the milk of term mothers.[66] These factors are thought to contribute to the higher IQ in preterm babies.

The variability of the fat content in breastmilk

Human milk-fat content has the widest degree of variability of any milk constituent, with considerable variation between mothers and in the same mother, as well as during feeds.

◆ The lowest fat content in breastmilk is found at the beginning of a feed, in the fore-milk.
◆ The highest fat content is found towards the end of a feed, in the hind-milk.

Opinion varies as to the exact increase in fat during the feed, but it is reported to be somewhere between double and treble.[49] Fat content also varies throughout the day: some studies have reported that it is lowest in the early morning and increases to its highest levels in early afternoon, while other studies reported the highest fat levels in the morning.[40]

Milk fat-content also varies with the stage of lactation. This may partly explain differences in the volume of breastmilk taken by healthy, term babies, for the total energy content of the milk may differ as the fat content varies. Therefore, it is suggested that milk with a high fat content may satisfy a baby sooner than milk with a low fat content. There is even the suggestion that appetite control may develop from the different fat levels between the fore-milk and hind-milk.[64]

Protein

Milk protein is of two types: casein and whey. Breastmilk is predominantly whey-based. This forms a softer gastric curd, thereby reducing gastric emptying time and aiding digestion.[67] Up to 90% of dietary protein can be used effectively by a baby.[67] Because absorption is efficient, less fat and protein are lost in the stools, consequently breastfed babies may pass stools less frequently than formula-fed babies.

In addition to proteins that provide nutrients, there are also non-nutritional proteins, such as anti-infective factors. It is the lactoglobulin fraction of the milk that contains the immunoglobulins previously mentioned in colostrum. These are produced in smaller quantities as the milk matures, but the increased volumes of breastmilk ensure that high levels of immunoglobulins are still available to the baby.[68]

Carbohydrate

Lactose is the main carbohydrate in breastmilk. Small amounts of galactose, fructose and oligosaccharides are also found. Lactose provides approximately 40% of the baby's energy needs. It not only enhances the absorption of calcium and iron, but is readily broken down to galactose and glucose. Glucose provides energy to the rapidly developing brain,[49] and galactose is needed in the development of the central nervous system.[67] Lactase, the enzyme necessary in the breakdown of lactose, is present in the intestinal mucosa from birth.

In the breastfed baby, lactose encourages the growth of *Lactobacillus bifidus* (*Bifidobacterium bifidum*) in the gut. Together, these work to keep the intestinal contents acid, thus inhibiting the growth of harmful bacteria.

The digestion of carbohydrate is helped by the enzyme amylase, which is normally found in the saliva and pancreatic juice of adults. In babies it is absent in saliva at birth and is present only in very small amounts in pancreatic juice; it is, however, present in breastmilk.

Water

Human milk is water-rich (approximately 87%). It has a low electrolyte concentration, which ensures sufficient free water is available, even when the weather is very hot or when a baby is in a tropical environment.[69]

Vitamins and minerals

The amounts of the fat-soluble vitamins A, D, E and K may vary in breastmilk according to its total fat content. Variations may similarly occur in the water-soluble vitamins, vitamin C, vitamin B complex and folic acid. Mothers who are vegans are at particular risk of vitamin deficiency, so too are mothers who are long-term users of oral contraceptives; both may particularly have a vitamin B_6 deficiency.[70] Vegan mothers, however, are usually careful in ensuring their diet is balanced.

High levels of vitamin K, which is important in the blood-clotting mechanism, are present in both colostrum and hind-milk;[70] a further reason why colostrum and hind-milk are important for all babies, especially those who are preterm and sick. This emphasizes the need to ensure that mothers who are expressing their milk begin as early as possible after birth. However, breastmilk is considered to contain insufficient vitamin K for the newborn, term baby during the first few days of life until he can produce his own. Insufficient vitamin K has been associated with haemorrhagic disease of the newborn. Studies appear to indicate that there is an increased risk of this condition in babies who are breastfed compared with those who are formula-fed.[71] Therefore, shortly after birth and with the parents' consent, prophylactic vitamin K is administered to all babies, either orally or by intramuscular injection, regardless of whether they are to receive breastmilk or formula. Extra doses may also be considered necessary for the sick and preterm baby.

Although rare, vitamin D deficiency in a baby may result in neonatal rickets.[72] This may be a problem, particularly if pregnant or breastfeeding women are deficient in vitamin D themselves.[73] Those most at risk of neonatal rickets are low-birthweight or preterm babies, and dark-skinned babies living in temperate climates where there may be little sunshine, especially during the winter months.[67] Supplements of calciferol (vitamin D) are commonly given to these babies when they receive breastmilk.

The levels of sodium, calcium, phosphorus and magnesium in breastmilk are considered ideal for the term, breastfed baby. However, this may not be the case for preterm babies (even though preterm breastmilk contains higher levels of these minerals). This is because their gastric and renal systems are immature, particularly in babies born before 32 weeks of gestation. Mineral supplementation of breastmilk to correct any deficiencies may be necessary. Hand-expression of breastmilk as opposed to mechanical expression (when expression is necessary) may be important in this context, for there is some evidence to suggest that this method of expression results in higher levels of some minerals, e.g. sodium.[74] It has been suggested that, while levels of minerals in formula milks have been artificially raised, absorption of these minerals may be more efficient in breastfed babies because of the presence of specific transport factors in breastmilk.

Trace elements

Iron is present in breastmilk in small amounts. A term baby, however, usually has sufficient stores of iron for at least the first 4–6 months, and is unlikely to require any supplements until solids are introduced.[75] The high levels of lactose and vitamin C in breastmilk help to facilitate iron absorption. The preterm baby, in contrast, may require iron supplementation because he is unable to absorb it effectively, and breastmilk may contain insufficient amounts for his needs.

Zinc is the most abundant trace mineral in human milk; its content is approximately eight times higher in colostrum than in mature milk, with a gradual decline as lactation progresses. Because it is important for growth, it is suggested that the higher levels in the early weeks of lactation reflect the higher growth velocity during this period.[76] Zinc is also essential to enzyme structure and function, and cellular immunity.

1.6 THE DEVELOPMENT OF A BABY'S FEEDING ABILITY

The ability of a baby to feed efficiently depends upon the coordination of the suck, swallow and breathing reflexes. The development of these reflexes begins during the fetal period and reaches maturity at approximately 40 weeks of gestation. Therefore, a term, healthy baby is usually well able to breastfeed soon after birth, while a preterm baby may take several days or weeks before this is possible. The question, to which there is still no really satisfactory answer, is, what kind of stimuli is most appropriate for a preterm baby, to help him learn to feed orally once outside the womb and which will also enhance the natural maturation process?

The following 'milestones' illustrate the normal developmental sequence of events leading to a term, healthy baby efficiently feeding at birth. This sequence has implications for helping a baby to 'learn' to breastfeed:

◆ At 8 weeks' gestation the fetus will respond to touch around the mouth area.
◆ Breathing movements can be seen on ultrasonography from 12 weeks' gestation.
◆ Oesophageal peristalsis and swallowing have been observed in the fetus from as early as 11 weeks in utero.[77]
◆ Taste is thought to develop around 12–15 weeks' gestation.
◆ Sucking (drawing something into the mouth) has been observed in various studies to begin between 18 weeks and 24 weeks.[78]
◆ Smell is considered to develop around 20 weeks' gestation.
◆ Hearing has been observed to begin around 20–24 weeks' gestation.
◆ Lingual and gastric lipases are detectable in the fetus from approximately 26 weeks' gestation.[59]

◆ The gag reflex is evident from 26–27 weeks in prematurely delivered babies.[78]

◆ Rooting, the response shown by a baby when touching the side of his cheek to encourage him to turn to the breast, with his mouth widely open, occurs around 32 weeks post-conception age.[78]

◆ A coordinated and effective use of the suck, swallow and breathing reflexes for nutritive purposes occurs at approximately 35–37 weeks post-conception age (though babies as young as 32 weeks are sometimes able to breastfeed efficiently).

A normal baby born at term, who is healthy, has a sufficiently mature suck and swallow reflex to breastfeed within a very short time of birth.[79]

1.6.1 The mother and the baby: breastfeeding at birth

Breastfeeding is an intricate and intimate relationship between a mother and her baby. Its success depends upon each working in synchrony with the other. Nature assists. As outlined above, the fetus develops its abilities to feed while still in the womb. During pregnancy the mother's breasts undergo changes which further aid feeding. They enlarge, as the glandular tissue becomes active and begins to fill with colostrum. The areolas may become larger, and may darken. On the surface of the areolas small pimple-like structures appear, called Montgomery's tubercles. These are sebaceous glands which secrete an oily fluid which keeps the skin in good condition, but in addition these secretions give the mothers' breasts their unique scent. The nipples may feel ultrasensitive. The mother may also notice an increase in the number of veins that criss-cross her breasts, an indication of the increased blood supply.

During normal labour and delivery both the mother and her baby experience huge rises in hormones of the adrenaline (epinephrine) family.[80] Contrary to popular belief, neither mother nor baby is sleepy after delivery (although they may be very tired); adrenaline (epinephrine) makes them both alert and acutely aware of each other's needs. It is at this time we can truly see what a baby is capable of doing. A term, healthy baby is born with an innate set of abilities specifically designed to ensure its survival. It can see, smell, taste, suck and swallow, touch, hear, and make positive whole body and hand-to-mouth movements. All of these have a crucial role in enabling a baby to breastfeed.

It is natural after birth for a mother to hold her newborn baby in her arms close to her breast. Observations made in Sweden show that even with the minimum of help, within 2 or so hours of delivery a term, healthy baby placed on his mother's abdomen is capable of finding the breast and feeding. The baby does this with a series of 'crawling' movements.[81]

The darkened areola and nipple are a visual marker for the baby; the scent from the Montgomery's glands in the areola is very attractive and encourages the baby to open his mouth widely and extend his tongue to taste the milk; not only does the baby move towards the nipple and areola but often touches the breast with his hand, helping to stimulate the release of prolactin, which produces milk, and oxytocin, which helps milk to flow. Human milk is slightly sweet in taste, which encourages a baby to use rhythmic sucking movements and continue feeding.

1.6.2 The normal pattern of suckling

The normal mature pattern of suckling begins with a period of quick sucking which stimulates the mother's let-down reflex. This is followed by a suck-swallow pattern which lasts for about 10–25 minutes. A mother should be able to hear her baby swallow. She may notice as the feed continues that he swallows with every one or two sucks, with the number of swallows decreasing towards the end of the feed.

The suck-swallow sequence is repeated approximately once a second. Each suck obtains approximately 0.2 mL of milk. The baby will continuously suck and swallow in 'bursts' of approximately 10 to 30 sucks with pauses in between. During these suck-swallow 'bursts' the baby also breathes, usually following the swallow. Suck-swallow rates may vary according to milk flow. During the pauses the lactiferous sinuses fill with milk. The pauses vary in length but are usually quite brief. It is thought that during these pauses the baby is able to recover from any respiratory compromise resulting from swallowing.

A premature baby may have only three to five sucks in each 'burst'. Breathing and swallowing occur before and after the bursts. Pauses between the 'bursts' may be equal to or much longer than the 'burst'.

1.6.3 Gestational age and the baby's natural breastfeeding ability

- ◆ Some well preterm babies as young as 28 weeks are able to lick milk expressed on to the nipple by the mother. The sweet taste encourages the baby to make rhythmic licking movements (Fig. 1.3).
- ◆ Up to 30 weeks post-conceptional age a baby is unlikely to receive his nutritive feeds orally. Most of his milk feeds will be given by gastric tube (and he may also require intravenous fluids).
- ◆ From approximately 30 weeks some babies can take small amounts of milk given orally.
- ◆ Between 30 weeks and 32 weeks, breastmilk can be given by cup or can be expressed directly into a baby's mouth, and he will be able to

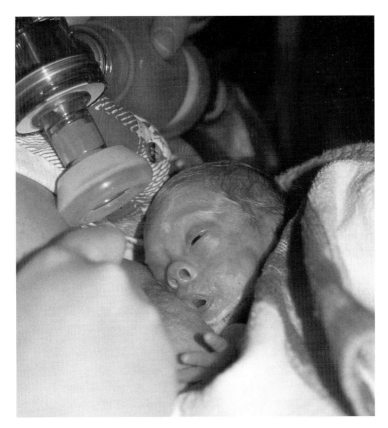

Figure 1.3 A well, preterm baby under 30 weeks about to taste his mother's milk.

lick milk from the nipple. Some babies may be able to attach at the breast although they may not yet begin to suckle, while others may suckle quite vigorously considering how young they are. For the majority of babies at this age, breastmilk will still be given mainly by gastric tube.

◆ From 32–34 weeks' gestation or post-conception age, gastric tube-feeding may still be important, but some babies will be able to take a complete breastfeed on one or several occasions over a 24-hour period. Most babies at this age will be able to cup-feed well and take appropriate amounts of fluid by this method.

◆ From 35 weeks onward, efficient breastfeeding is possible.

◆ By 37 weeks' gestation or post-conception age a well baby is usually able to sustain his nutrition totally at the breast.

1.7 FACTORS AFFECTING A BABY'S ABILITY TO FEED EFFICIENTLY

A number of conditions may affect a baby's ability to feed efficiently. These may be physical, neurological, chromosomal, metabolic or clinical in origin.

Physical problems that affect the mechanics of feeding include:

◆ cleft lip and/or palate
◆ a very high curved palate, which can occur in preterm babies who have been ventilated for a long period (although oral plates may prevent or reduce the likelihood of this occurring)
◆ a short frenulum to the tongue (tongue-tie)
◆ a protruding or large tongue, which is a feature in some babies with Down's syndrome
◆ a small and receding lower jaw and a short tongue, as in Pierre Robin syndrome.

Other physical conditions that do not affect the baby's ability to feed orally but affect the overall efficiency of feeding include pyloric stenosis (a narrowing of the muscular wall of the pylorus between the stomach and the jejunum).

While there is no doubt that some of these conditions may interfere with efficient oral feeding, breastfeeding may be easier to establish and be more successful than bottle-feeding. If a mother has an efficient let-down reflex, the baby may be able to obtain sufficient quantities of milk without having to expend excessive energy or physical effort.

The coordination of the suck, swallow and breathing reflexes may be compromised by extreme prematurity or illness (causing the baby to be weak). For apparently healthy babies of at least 36 weeks' gestation or post-conception age whose reflexes do not appear to be well coordinated, the reasons may be more difficult to identify. These babies are commonly among those admitted to neonatal or paediatric units with 'feeding problems' within the first few days after delivery. One explanation may be that some term babies naturally take several days to develop a mature sucking pattern and that it is not uncommon for 1 or 2 days to elapse before a mature pattern emerges. It also appears that the lower the gestational age of the baby, the longer the period required to develop a mature pattern of sucking, so that it may take a baby of 32 weeks up to 6–8 weeks to show a mature pattern.[82]

Maternal analgesia or sedation used during labour may affect a baby's readiness to feed, and his level of arousal. Pethidine has certainly been implicated in babies failing to feed efficiently in the first few days after birth.[83]

Babies with a neurological condition frequently have problems coordinating their suck, swallow and breathing reflexes. They may have a number of symptoms which interfere with their ability to feed by any conventional method.[84] These include:

◆ a weak suck, swallow and gag reflex
◆ an abnormal tongue movement
◆ a sucking movement that shows no regular pattern
◆ an abnormal 'biting' action
◆ flaccid muscle tone of the mouth and head (and of the whole body)
◆ excessive arching of the body.

Babies with respiratory and cardiac problems tire easily, and use more energy to maintain respiration and circulation. They usually gain weight slowly regardless of how they are fed. Increasing the volume of breastmilk to ensure adequate nutrient and energy content may not be possible because the volume required may be too great or, during the acute or chronic phase of the condition, the baby may be fluid-restricted and need a nutrient/energy-dense supplement.

Certain metabolic disorders may make breastfeeding and the use of expressed breastmilk impossible. These include rare conditions in which there is a primary deficiency of lactase, the enzyme vital in the breakdown of lactose. Galactosaemia, for example, affects the metabolism of lactose, because the liver enzyme galactose is missing. Such conditions become very obvious in the first weeks of life but fortunately are uncommon.

The mother's 'natural' nipple shape may affect a baby's attachment at the breast. Flat or inverted nipples, for example, may be more difficult for a preterm or weak baby to draw effectively into his mouth to form a long 'teat' of breast tissue. A long or a very large and fibrous nipple, in contrast, may make correct attachment difficult to achieve because the baby, particularly if preterm, has too much tissue in his mouth and cannot reach the lactiferous sinuses effectively, and in addition the tissue may not be soft enough. Attention to attachment and positioning is critical in these situations.

REFERENCES

1. Williams AF (1993) Human milk and the preterm baby. *Lancet* **306**: 1628–1629.
2. Whiteley W (1996) A parent's experience of a special care baby unit. Emotional dimensions of prematurity. *Prof Care Mother Child* **6**: 141–142.
3. Helsing E, King FS (1982) *Breast-feeding in Practice: A Manual for Health Workers*. Oxford: Oxford University Press, p. 178.

4. World Health Organization (1984) Infant feeding: the physiological basis. *WHO Bull* (suppl.) **67**: 30–31.

5. World Health Organization (1993) Global breast-feeding prevalence and trends. In: *Breast-feeding: The Technical Basis and Recommendations for Action.* Saadeh RJ, Labock MH, Cooney KA, Koniz-Booher P (eds). Geneva: WHO, pp. 1–19.

6. World Health Organization (1997) *Improving Child Health. IMCI: the integrated approach.* WHO/CHD97.12 Geneva: WHO.

7. Department of Health (1995) *Breastfeeding: Good Practice Guidance to the NHS.*

8. Singhal A, Cole TJ, Lucas A (2001) Early nutrition in preterm infants and later blood pressure: two cohorts after randomised trials. *Lancet* **357**: 406–407.

9. Oddy WH, Holt PG, Sly PD et al (1999) Association between breastfeeding and asthma in 6 year old children: findings of a prospective birth cohort study. *BMJ* **319**: 815–819.

10. Wilson AC, Forsyth JS, Greene SA et al (1998) Relation of infant diet to childhood health: seven year follow up of cohort of children in Dundee infant feeding study. *BMJ* **316**: 21–25.

11. Lucas A, Cole TJ (1990) Breastmilk and necrotising enterocolitis. *Lancet* **336**: 1519–1523.

12. Howie PJ, Forsyth J, Ogston SA et al (1990) Protective effect of breastfeeding against infection. *BMJ* **300**: 11–16.

13. La Leche League (1999) *Breastfeeding and Dental Health* [information leaflet reviewing evidence]. London: LLLGB.

14. Labbock MH, Henderson GE (1987) Does breastfeeding protect against malocclusion? *Am J Prev* **3**: 227.

15. Saarinen UM (1982) Prolonged breastfeeding as prophylaxis for recurrent otitis media. *Acta Paediatr Scand* **3**: 227–232.

16. Williamson IG, Dunleavey J, Robinson D (1994) Risk factors in otitis media with effusion. A 1 year case control study in 5–7 year old children. *Fam Pract* **11**: 271–274.

17. Park P (1992) Cows' milk linked to juvenile diabetes. *New Scientist* **1835**: 9 (22 August).

18. Karjalainen I, Martin JM, Knip M (1992) A bovine albumin peptide as a possible trigger of insulin-dependent diabetes mellitus. *N Engl J Med* **327**: 302–307.

19. Lucas A, Cole TJ (1990) Breastmilk and neonatal necrotising enterocolitis. *Lancet* **336**: 1519–1521.

20. Shu XO, Clemens J, Zheng W et al (1995) Infant breastfeeding and the risk of childhood lymphoma and leukemia. *Int J Epidemiol* **24**: 27–32.

21. Matthew DJ, Taylor B, Norman AP et al (1977) Prevention of eczema. *Lancet* **i**: 321–324.

22. Lucas A, Morley R, Cole TJ et al (1992) Breastmilk and subsequent intelligence quotient in children born preterm. *Lancet* **339**: 261–264.

23. Farquharson J, Cockburn F, Patrick WA et al (1992) Infant cerebral cortex phospholipid fatty-acid composition and diet. *Lancet* **340**: 810–813.

24. Paradise JL, Elster BA, Tan L (1994) Evidence in infants with cleft palate that breastmilk protects against otitis media. *Pediatrics* **94**: 853–860.

25. Broad FE (1972) The effects of infant feeding on speech quality. *NZ Med J* **76**: 28–31.

26. Newcomb PA, Storer BE, Longnecker MP et al (1994) Lactation and a reduced risk of premenopausal breast cancer. *N Engl J Med* **330**: 81–87.
27. Reuter K, Baker SP, Krolikowski FJ (1992) Risk factors for breast cancer in women undergoing mammography. *Am J Roentgenol* **158**: 273–278.
28. Yoo KY, Tajima K, Kuroishi T et al (1992) Independent protective effect of lactation against breast cancer: a case-control study in Japan. *Am J Epidemiol* **135**: 726–733.
29. Cummings RG, Klineberg RJ (1993) Breastfeeding and other reproductive factors and the risk of hip fracture in elderly women. *Int J Epidemiol* **2**: 684–691.
30. Elsman J (1998) Relevance of pregnancy and lactation to osteoporosis. *Lancet* **352**: 504.
31. Gross B (1991) Is the lactational amenorrhea method a part of natural family planning? Biology and policy. *Am J Obstet Gynecol* **165**: 2014–2019.
32. Lewis PR, Brown JB, Renfrew MB et al (1991) The resumption of ovulation and menstruation in a well-nourished population of women breastfeeding for an extended period of time. *Fertil Steril* **55**: 529–536.
33. Dugdale AE, Eaton-Evans J (1989) The effect of lactation and other factors on post-partum changes in body-weight and triceps skinfold thickness. *Br J Nutr* **61**: 149–153.
34. Saadeh RJ, ed. (1993) *Breastfeeding: The Technical Basis and Recommendations for Action.* Geneva: WHO.
35. World Health Organization (2001) The optimal duration of exclusive breastfeeding. Results of a WHO systematic review. Press release No. 7, 2 April 2001.
36. World Health Organization (1989) Infant feeding: the physiological basis. *WHO Bull* (suppl.) **67**: 20.
37. World Health Organization (1989) Infant feeding: the physiological basis. *WHO Bull* (suppl.) **67**: 21.
38. Madden JD, Boyar RM, MacDonald PC et al (1997) Analysis of secretory patterns of prolactin and gonadotrophins during twenty-four hours in a lactating woman before and after resumption of menses. *Am J Obstet Gynecol* **132**: 436.
39. Wilde CJ, Prentice A, Peaker M (1995) Breastfeeding: matching supply and demand in human lactation. *Proc Nutr Soc* **54**: 401–406.
40. Lammi-Keefe CJ, Ferris AM, Jensen RG (1990) Changes in human milk at 0600, 1000, 1400, 1800, and 2200 h. *J Pediatr Gastroent Nutr* **11**: 83–88.
41. Burman D (1982) Nutrition in early childhood. In: *Nutrition in Growth and Development*, Part I. *Textbook of Paediatric Nutrition*, 2nd edn. McLaren D, Burman D (eds). Edinburgh: Churchill Livingstone, pp. 39–72.
42. Gross SJ, David RJ, Bauman L et al (1980) Nutritional composition of milk produced by mothers delivering preterm. *J Pediatr* **96**: 641–644.
43. Silber GH, Hachey DL, Schanler RJ et al (1988) Manipulation of maternal diet to alter fatty acid composition of human milk intended for premature infants. *Am J Clin Nutr* **47**: 810–814.
44. Specker BL (1994) Nutritional concerns of lactating women consuming vegetarian diets. *Am J Clin Nutr* **59** (suppl.): 1182–1186S.
45. Wallace JP, Inbar G, Ernsthausen K (1992) Infant acceptance of postexercise breastmilk. *Pediatrics* **89**: 1245–1247.
46. Neville MC (1995) Volume and caloric density of human milk. In: *Handbook of Milk Composition.* Jensen RG (ed.). San Diego: Academic Press, p. 101.

47. Butte NE, Villapando S, Wong WW et al (1992) Human milk intake and growth faltering of rural Mesoamerindian infants. *Am J Clin Nutr* **55**: 1109.

48. Kunz C, Rodriguez-Palmero M, Koletzko B et al (1999) Nutritional and biochemical properties of human milk, Part 1. General aspects, proteins and carbohydrates. In: *Clinics in Perinatology. Clinical Aspects of Human Milk and Lactation.* Wagner C, Purohit DM (eds). London: Saunders.

49. Jelliffe DB, Jelliffe EFP (1978) Biochemical considerations. In: *Human Milk in the Modern World.* Oxford: Oxford University Press, p. 28.

50. Odent M (1990) The unknown human infant. *J Hum Lact* **6**: 6–8.

51. Jannson L, Karlson FA, Westermark B (1985) Mitogenic activity and epidermal growth factor content in human milk. *Acta Paediatr Scand* **74**: 250–253.

52. Carpenter G (1980) Epidermal growth factor is a major growth-promoting agent in human milk. *Science* **210**: 198–199.

53. De Carvalho M, Klaus MH, Merkatz RB (1982) Frequency of breast-feeding and serum bilirubin. *Am J Dis Child* **136**: 737–738.

54. Cure in a mother's milk. *New Scientist* 20 April 1991.

55. Mathur NB, Dwarkadas AM, Sharma VK et al (1990) Anti-infective factors in preterm human colostrum. *Acta Paediatr Scand* **79**: 1039–1044.

56. Reissland N, Burghart R (1988) The quality of a mothers milk and the health of her child: beliefs and practices of the women of Mithila. *Soc Sci Med* **27**: 461–469.

57. Hamosh M, Bitman J, Fink CS et al (1985) Lipid composition of preterm human milk and its digestion by the infant. In: *Composition and Physiological Properties of Human Milk.* Schaub J (ed.). Oxford: Elsevier, pp. 153–164.

58. Steichen JJ, Krug-Wispe SK, Tsang RC (1987) Breastfeeding the low birth weight infant. *Clin Perinatol* **14**: 1.

59. Hamosh M (1987) Lipid metabolism in premature infants. *Biol Neonate* **52** (suppl.): 50–64.

60. Hamosh M (1979) A review. Fat digestion in the newborn: role of lingual lipase and preduodenal digestion. *Pediatr Res* **13**: 615–622.

61. Hernell O, Blackberg L (1988) Lipolysis in human milk: causes and consequences. In: *Composition and Physiological Properties of Human Milk.* Schaub J (ed.). Oxford: Elsevier, pp. 165–178.

62. Freed LM, Neville MC, Hamosh M (1986) Diurnal and within-feed variations in lipase activity and triglyceride content of human milk. *J Pediatr Gastroenterol Nutr* **5**: 938–942.

63. Canadian Paediatric Society Committee on Nutrition (1981) Feeding the low birth weight infant. *Can Med Assoc* **124**: 1301–1311.

64. Jackson KA, Gibson RA (1989) Weaning foods cannot replace breastmilk as sources of long-chain polyunsaturated fatty acids. *Am J Clin Nutr* **50**: 980–982.

65. Nettleton JA (1993) Are n-3 fatty acids essential nutrients for fetal and infant development? *J Am Diet Assoc* **93**: 58–64.

66. Ghebremeskel K, Leighfield M (1992) Infant brain lipids and diet [letter]. *Lancet* **340**: 1093.

67. World Health Organization (1989) Infant feeding: the physiological basis. *WHO Bull* **67** (suppl.): 25–26.

68. Jatsyk GV, Kuvaeva IB, Gribakin SG (1985) Immunological protection of the neonatal gastrointestinal tract: the importance of breastfeeding. *Acta Paediatr Scand* **74**: 246–249.

69. Almroth S, Bidinger PD (1990) No need for water supplementation for exclusively breast-fed infants under hot and arid conditions. *Trans Roy Soc Trop Med Hygiene* **84**: 602–604.

70. World Health Organization (1989) Infant feeding: the physiological basis. *WHO Bull* **67** (suppl.): 28–29.

71. McNinch AW, Tripp JH (1991) Haemorrhagic disease of the newborn in the British Isles: two-year prospective study. *BMJ* **303**: 1105–1109.

72. Chang YT, Germain-Lee EL, Doran TF et al (1992) Hypocalcaemia in non-white breast-fed infants. *Clin Pediatr* **31**: 695–698.

73. Rothberg AD, Pettifor JM, Cohen DF et al (1982) Maternal-infant vitamin D relationships during breast-feeding. *J Pediatr* **101**: 500–503.

74. Lang S, Lawrence CJ, L'E Orme R (1994) Sodium in hand and pump expressed human breastmilk. *Early Hum Dev* **38**: 131–138.

75. DHSS (1991) *Present Day Practice in Infant Feeding: Third Report*, 4th edn. London: HMSO.

76. Riordan J (1993) The biologic specificity of breastmilk. In: *Breastfeeding and Human Lactation*. Riordan J, Auerbach KG (eds). London: Jones & Bartlett, pp. 105–129.

77. Lebenthal E, Heitlinger L, Milla PJ (1988) Prenatal and perinatal development of the gastrointestinal tract. In *Harries' Paediatric Gastroenterology*, 2nd edn. Milla PJ, Muller DPR (eds). Edinburgh: Churchill Livingstone.

78. McBride MC, Danner SC (1987) Sucking disorders in neurologically impaired infants: assessment and facilitation of breastfeeding. *Clin Perinatol* **14**: 109–130.

79. Widstrom AM, Thingstrom-Pausson J (1993) The position of the tongue during rooting reflexes elicited in newborn infants before the first suckle. *Acta Paediatr Scand* **82**: 281–283.

80. Odent M (1987) The fetus ejection reflex. *Birth* **14**: 104–105.

81. Widstrom AM (1996) *Breastfeeding: The Baby's Choice* [Video]. Ace Graphics, http://www.acegraphics.com.au.

82. Meyer Palmer M, Crawley K, Blanco IA (1993) Neonatal oral-motor assessment scale: a reliability study. *J Perinatol* **8**: 30–35.

83. Righard L, Alade MO (1990) Effect of delivery room routines on success of first breast-feed. *Lancet* **336**: 1105–1107.

84. La Leche League International (1992) The neurologically impaired baby. In: *The Breastfeeding Answer Book*, vol. 15. Schaumburg, Ill: LLLI, pp. 336–337.

2

The position and attachment of the baby at the breast

2.1 POSITIONING AND BREAST ATTACHMENT

This chapter is primarily about the positioning and breast attachment of babies who have special needs: they may be small, have low energy reserves, be clinically unwell, have temporarily or permanently impaired oral function, or quite simply their feeding reflexes may be uncoordinated in the first few hours or days after delivery.[1] Any mother who wishes to breastfeed her baby – and it does not matter whether it is within minutes, hours or weeks after birth – has, with her baby, to acquire the key skills of positioning and attachment. These skills are crucial not only to the success of breastfeeding but also to the maintenance of healthy breasts and nipples. What is perhaps little appreciated is that 'positioning' is the skill the mother has to develop, while 'attachment' is the skill the baby has to develop. Although each skill is independently acquired, breastfeeding only succeeds when the mother and baby have both mastered them equally well.

When considering babies who need 'special care', it is frequently the case that the skills are acquired over different time periods. It is not unusual, for example, for the mother to acquire the skill of positioning some time before her baby develops the ability to use the skill of attachment to remove milk efficiently from the mother's breast. Therefore, in this chapter, positioning is discussed before attachment.

No two mother-and-baby pairs will breastfeed in exactly the same way, with respect to where the mother is most comfortable, what position the baby is in, the mother's anatomy, and so on. Many of the images mothers see of breastfeeding in videos, pictures and in some books lead them to suppose they must sit in a chair and hold their baby across their chest. This impression is commonly reinforced by their experience in hospital. However, go into mothers' homes and very quickly it is apparent that circumstances and personal preferences make breastfeeding a creative activity which is unique to each mother and baby. A wealth of possible positions for either the baby or the mother to enable breastfeeding to happen are being tried, discovered and experimented with. In a neonatal unit where a mother may face more challenges than normal in the techniques of breastfeeding, perhaps we should be more adventurous and introduce mothers to the possibilities that exist, thus increasing the likelihood of success for any mother who wants to breastfeed.

The only real 'rules' for positioning and attachment are given as 'key points'; beyond these, this chapter aims to give as many options as possible to make it possible to help any mother and baby, in any situation in a neonatal unit (and elsewhere) to breastfeed.

2.1.1 How long will it take to acquire the skills necessary for breastfeeding?

The length of time needed to acquire the skills of positioning and attachment will vary according to the mother's natural ability, her physical condition after delivery, the baby's condition at birth, his level of maturity, and any physical or other problems which may be present. The majority of healthy, term babies can breastfeed within 1–2 hours of birth without any difficulties. A very small number of these babies may have a delay of 1–2 days and sometimes even longer before their suck, swallow and breathing reflexes are coordinated well enough to breastfeed effectively. These babies frequently appear on special care baby units because they have feeding problems for which no real cause can be found, and given a little time they appear to recover with no aftereffects. In other words, there is a natural time 'window' during which the reflexes necessary for effective feeding mature and become coordinated – and this will vary slightly from baby to baby.

The developmental stages through which a preterm (and therefore an immature) baby passes in order to effectively breastfeed are programmed to occur in a particular sequence, resulting in the behaviour outlined in Table 2.1. Some preterm babies will naturally progress along the developmental pathway more quickly than others. This may depend on how well he is. The gestational ages listed in Table 2.1 are for guidance only; if a baby has a stable heart rate and is able to breathe without difficulty, and is generally well, he should have the opportunity to begin the learning process for breastfeeding irrespective of gestational age or weight.[2] Each baby will pass through these developmental 'time windows' at a different speed, and no amount of trying to make a baby breastfeed before he is ready will work. As a rule of thumb, it is better to tell parents not to expect their preterm baby to breastfeed efficiently before the approximate date that he would have been born (though in many cases a preterm baby will fully breastfeed much earlier than this).

A term baby who is ill at birth or shortly afterwards may be developmentally able to breastfeed but may not have the energy to do so and

Table 2.1 A preterm baby's normal behaviour at the breast at different gestations or levels of maturity

Gestational age	At the breast a baby can:
Level 1 Less than 30 weeks	Smell; open his mouth; protrude his tongue; dribble saliva; lick milk from the nipple; take some breast tissue into his mouth; make a few weak sucks
Level 2 30–32 weeks	As above; can also attach to the breast. MAY make some weak to strong sucks with long pauses in between
Level 3 32 + weeks	As above; MAY root; organize sucking bursts with long pauses; take part of a feed from the breast; take one to all complete feeds from the breast
Level 4 36 + weeks	As above; can also breastfeed in a well-coordinated way

may show immature feeding behaviour reminiscent of preterm babies. Babies with neurological damage may require several weeks or even months before they are able to breastfeed efficiently. In some cases the level of damage to the brain is such that the baby may never be able to breastfeed effectively, and the small number of babies who have a poor or absent gag reflex are unlikely to feed orally.

To breastfeed, a baby HAS to respond to the breast in a certain predictable way, and all babies will go through at least part of the sequence illustrated in Box 2.1, although the timing of this will vary. A baby who is stressed or compromised in some way may not behave in a way expected for his gestational age. A term baby with tachypnoea of the newborn, for example, may go from being in an incubator, to simply lying close to the breast but not having enough energy to breastfeed, to effective feeding, in a few hours or within 1–2 days. A baby who is severely birth-asphyxiated may take several weeks or even months to go through these stages.

Irrespective of what the problem is, any baby who responds to the breast in a predictable way at some point in the sequence outlined in Box 2.1, i.e by opening his mouth in response to the smell of his mother's breast and who puts his tongue out to lick the nipple, and can take breastmilk onto his tongue and swallow it, can obtain some or all of his nutrition at the breast, or he can at the very least show his mother that her milk is special to him from the way he reacts. The question is, what are the expectations of the mother and of those who care for her?

> **Box 2.1** The sequential behaviour of any baby at the breast, which may lead to breastfeeding.
>
> To breastfeed, a baby:
>
> ◆ smells the breast
> ◆ may become more alert and look at the breast
> ◆ opens his mouth
> ◆ may 'root' for the breast
> ◆ protrudes his tongue, may dribble
> ◆ may lick milk from the nipple
> ◆ may take breast tissue into his mouth
> ◆ may suck weakly or strongly
> ◆ may audibly swallow
> ◆ develops organized sucking bursts
> ◆ may have short or very long pauses between sucks
> ◆ may touch the breast with his fingers

Unrealistic expectations of what a baby can do may lead to a mother feeling that she is a failure, to disappointment, to feeling that her baby is not interested in breastfeeding, or even that her baby is not developing normally. Those caring for the baby have to be careful not to use language which makes these feelings even more pronounced. For example, to ask a mother of a preterm baby of 32 weeks' gestation if her baby 'has had a good breastfeed', or to suggest that the mother 'tries to breastfeed' is guaranteed to make the mother feel that either she or her baby have failed. Mothers of babies in neonatal and paediatric units, and those of us who care for them, have to consider how she wishes to eventually feed her baby. Breastfeeding may be the goal; but for many babies in our care that may not be immediately possible. It is crucial therefore to be able to break down into achievable stages how that goal will be reached, and to discuss these with the mother and her family.

2.2 THE PRACTICAL ASPECTS OF POSITIONING AND ATTACHMENT

There is no one correct position for breastfeeding. A mother has several options to choose from, depending upon her and her baby's needs.

Attachment, in contrast, has to be exact if it is going to result in the baby obtaining milk. The two skills are the fundamental keys to successful breastfeeding – the time and patience spent helping a mother and her baby in the early days will be remembered long after the mother has left the unit.

On one hand a neonatal unit is a technological wonderworld, particularly if it is where you work; on the other hand, if *your* baby is admitted to one it will seem initially a 'shocking' environment, full of complex-looking machinery, alarms, buzzers, busy, busy staff and bright lights.

Breastfeeding is an intimate interaction between a mother and her baby, and the environment in which she learns to feed (or express her breastmilk) can greatly influence her success. It is important to understand how the woman feels when revealing her breasts, particularly in the early days, how nervous she is, how tense she may feel, and how worried she is that someone may interrupt her, or watch what she is doing.

2.2.1 Before assisting a mother with positioning and attaching her baby to the breast

Ensure privacy, particularly in the initial period while the mother and baby are learning what to do. This may be achieved simply by using screens, or even by turning the mother's chair away from other people in a quiet part of a unit or a room set aside for this purpose. Conversely, breastfeeding should not be something a mother feels she has to 'hide away' to do in private. She should feel that she can feed discreetly anywhere she chooses. Therefore, what she wears, and how confident she is in her ability to breastfeed, are very important. A neonatal unit can be a positive 'training' environment for a mother to learn how to breastfeed, giving her time to develop the necessary skills and to become comfortable feeding when other people are around.

The mother needs to be comfortable either on a bed, in a chair or on the floor. If she is in a chair, it should:

◆ be wide enough for both the mother and baby to be relaxed
◆ be low enough for the mother's feet to be flat on the floor and for her lap to be flat (crossing her legs is an unstable position for any length of time and can become very uncomfortable; if the chair is too high for the mother to keep her lap flat, she should rest her feet on a firm pillow, a stool, or a pile of books such as telephone directories)
◆ have arm rests on which the mother can support her arms; this helps her to support her baby (Fig. 2.1)
◆ have a firm, high back for support and to lean against.

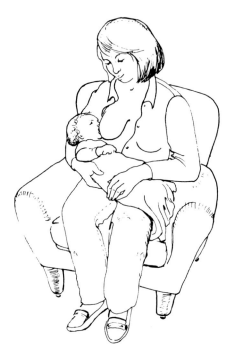

Figure 2.1 An ideal nursing chair.

While a rocking chair may be comfortable and relaxing once the establishment of breastfeeding has taken place, it may not provide enough stability for the mother and baby when they are both learning to breastfeed.

If the mother is on a bed or on the floor:

◆ she will require sufficient soft pillows around her for firm, comfortable support
◆ she may find two or three soft pillows placed under her knees adds to her comfort and stability (Fig. 2.2)
◆ if she is lying on her side she may find a pillow under her waist is comfortable
◆ a pillow under her chest and shoulders may help her to position her breasts, if they are large or long, so that her baby is able to take more breast tissue into his mouth (see Fig. 2.10)
◆ she can lean against the wall, head of the bed or against the sofa or chair.

The mother's clothing should be practical: for example, blouses or dresses with buttons down the front, or loose T-shirt style tops. A hair

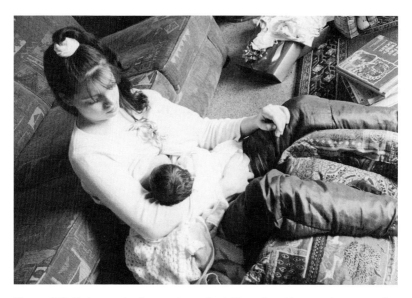

Figure 2.2 Sitting on the floor to breastfeed. Note the ribbon used to tie up the mother's sweater.

clip, a bulldog clip or a peg is useful for holding clothing away from the mother's breast, so that she does not have to support her clothes with her hand (Fig. 2.3). Alternatively, one end of a piece of ribbon may be passed through the neck of a T-shirt or sweater, looped under the hem and then tied to the other end at the neck, so that her clothing does not cover the breast and her hands are free (see Fig. 2.2). The brassière or upper garment must not be tight around the margins of the breast or restrict access to the nipple area, as this may prevent efficient drainage of the milk, resulting in a blocked duct or lobe. Brassières that open in the front are useful. Soft sports brassières are comfortable, particularly for small breasts which do not become uncomfortably heavy. A brassière does not have to be worn, however. The mother should wear whatever is most comfortable for her and can be unfastened or loosened easily for breastfeeding to take place.

A preterm baby – particularly one less than 35 weeks – may benefit from being lightly wrapped for a breastfeed. This reduces the amount of stimulation the baby receives through moving his arms, which may distract him from his feeding experience. A term baby does not need to be wrapped up to breastfeed, though some mothers may find it easier to feed when the baby's arms are not in the way. It is not unusual to observe a term, healthy baby touching or stroking his mother's breasts

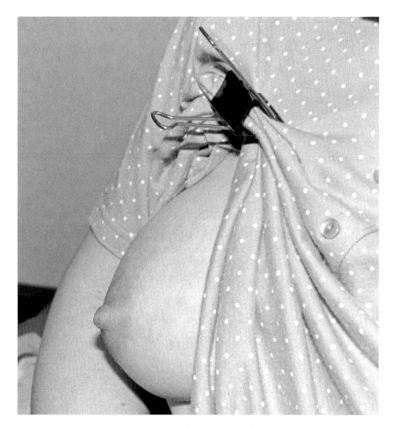

Figure 2.3 A method of securing clothing to make breastfeeding easier.

before or during a feed. Although it has not been fully researched, it may be beneficial for the baby to do this. If the nipple is touched it may be stimulated to become more erect and thus enhance attachment. In addition, though not necessarily physiologically related, the tactile stimulation of the baby fingering the mother's nipple and areola may encourage the release of the hormones prolactin and oxytocin and thereby aid an efficient milk flow – in effect the baby can 'call up' the milk.

Small blankets, towels and soft pillows can all be used to support the baby; these can be positioned easily by the mother without help. They need to be on a table or stool placed near enough to the mother to be within her easy reach. Larger pillows can be too bulky for this purpose and are more difficult for the mother to put in the right place when she is on her own.

A cold or warm drink should be available within easy reach of the mother … and maybe a couple of digestive biscuits? Beware of very hot fluids – they can cause burns.

Finally, it is important that if you are helping a mother you have enough time to spend with her and, if your help is practical, that you too are sitting comfortably on a small chair or stool. If you stoop to help her you risk damaging your own back.

2.2.2 What is meant by positioning?

Breastfeeding depends upon a mother being able to position or hold her baby in such a way that he can easily reach the nipple and areola, and take sufficient breast tissue into his mouth to ensure the lactiferous sinuses are inside and not outside his mouth – and on the mother being able to maintain that position until her baby has finished his feed. Sometimes it is not quite so straightforward. It does not **only** mean the mother physically picking her baby up and positioning him in her arms, it may also mean the mother positioning herself – her body – in relation to her baby so that breastfeeding can easily take place, for example positions where the mother is leaning over her baby. This will be seen more clearly later on in the chapter in the discussion of less conventional breastfeeding positions.

We should emphasize that 'positioning' is much more than simply a way of facilitating breastfeeding. It is also about closeness, security, warmth, comfort and reassurance, and for the mothers, it is part of the 'healing' process which takes place after having a baby admitted to a special care unit. It is these factors that make it so very important for the mothers of babies needing special care, who may still have to wait for breastfeeding to take place.

Maintaining a breastfeeding position

Whatever position the mother adopts to feed her baby, she has to be able to maintain it for at least 20–40 minutes. Little adjustment can be made to the original position once the baby is attached and suckling at the breast. This may sound obvious, but the reality is that many mothers do not realize how long they will have to hold or support their baby, or how heavy any baby can be after the first few minutes! It can be useful if mothers have some idea of this before they breastfeed a baby in special care, for these babies are the ones who are least able to deal with suboptimal positioning and attachment. It can be useful to have one or two very simple cloth dolls filled with beans and polystyrene weighing around 2–3 kg (5–7 lb). Mothers can use these to practise positioning and maintaining the position. These dolls are very simple and cheap to make.

How to support a baby to breastfeed

It is common to assume that 'positioning' a baby also requires some kind of support. A pillow is frequently given to mothers in hospital; but there are many other ways to support a baby. **What** to use will be influenced by:

◆ the baby's size
◆ his condition
◆ the baby's breastfeeding position
◆ the size of the mother's breasts
◆ where the mother feeds.

There are many ways a mother can support her baby so that he can maintain his attachment at the breast. These include using:

◆ the arms of the chair
◆ a stool or books
◆ soft pillows or cushions
◆ towels, blankets, etc.
◆ the mother's lap
◆ her arms
◆ sitting cross-legged
◆ a hard surface such as a table, the floor or a bed.

The position the mother adopts to feed will influence the type of support she will find useful.

Sitting positions

If the mother is sitting in a chair:

◆ She may find that resting her arms on the arms of the chair is sufficient.
◆ If her baby is small, a towel or small blanket can be tucked into the place where support is needed to keep the baby in the right position.
◆ Putting one foot on a stool or pile of books may raise one leg sufficiently above lap height for the mother to rest her arm and the baby against her thigh. The baby should then be high enough to easily reach the mother's nipple and areola. This is useful for a small baby.
◆ The mother's lap should be flat; a stool or books under her feet may be needed to ensure this. If the mother needs to lie her baby flat on her lap so that she can lean over to feed him, she may need a table in front of her with a soft pillow on the edge to lean her head on. She may need a thin pillow on her lap or a folded towel or blanket to raise the baby sufficiently to reach the breast. If the breasts are large she may need nothing in her lap.

If the mother is sitting on the floor or on a bed:

◆ She can sit cross-legged. Her thighs support her arms and the 'hollow' she has created between her legs is an ideal shape for her to support her baby's bottom. Sitting cross-legged the mother often needs no other means of support for the baby.
◆ She may need pillows behind her back or under her knees (Fig. 2.2).

Leaning positions

If the mother is using a leaning position:

◆ She may need to support her head on a pillow laid on the edge of the table.
◆ The baby may lie on the bed, or on a blanket or pillow on the floor.

Lying positions

If the mother is lying down:

◆ She may appreciate soft pillows, particularly to protect a new scar from a caesarean section.
◆ A small towel or blanket may be useful for her to 'wedge' her baby into a good position, so that he can maintain his attachment.

How to get started

The mother and her partner should be encouraged to have as much contact with their baby as possible. The mother in particular needs to become accustomed to holding her baby in her arms next to her breast, to cuddling him, to touching him, to letting him hear the comforting beat of her heart. The more she is used to touching him and holding him the more confident she will become, and the more relaxed and easier breastfeeding will be. Initially both she and her partner may need considerable encouragement to hold their baby, but as long as he is stable it will cause him no distress, indeed it may be beneficial to all the family. This kind of closeness can begin even if the baby is ventilated and very preterm, providing he is stable. Several studies show how much babies benefit from this closeness, particularly when the contact is skin-to-skin.[3] In some ways it can be a bonus to have the time to spend getting used to holding a baby without having the pressure to breastfeed him immediately he is born. Even if the mother has this opportunity only for a short time on the day of birth, it will help to give her confidence when she later assists her baby in attaching to the breast for the first time. This is particularly true of mothers who have given birth to preterm babies before they were able to attend any antenatal classes, or indeed mothers who were not planning to attend antenatal classes. In both cases those mothers are unlikely to know the key points of positioning and attachment.

A mother should not, initially, feel under pressure from anyone to hold her baby next to her skin – although if she is willing to do so it should definitely be encouraged. As she becomes more used to holding him, skin contact should be suggested and encouraged in as private and relaxed an environment as is possible.

During the time the mother is growing used to holding her baby she can be given information about the positioning options for breastfeeding. If the baby is stable and at rest she can practise holding him in different ways as described below. If she is staying in the unit (or in the maternity unit), or if there is a spare bed, she can practise lying-down positions. If her baby is not stable but the mother is receptive to learning about positioning she can practise using a doll. Sometimes it can be fun to get a group of mothers together to practise different positions using dolls – humour can be a valuable aid to helping mothers relax, and group work gives them mutual support and solidarity. Giving the mother the opportunity to try different positions, and find ones which she is comfortable using *before* her baby begins to breastfeed, or at times when her baby is resting, can greatly increase her confidence.

2.2.3 The mother's anatomy and positioning

Each mother's breasts are different in size, in shape, in the way they protrude from the chest wall, the direction they fall in, the size and shape of the areola, and of the nipple. These differences subtly affect the way a baby is positioned for breastfeeding, and few mothers will hold their babies for breastfeeding in exactly the same way. It may seem rather bizarre to suggest to a mother that when she is alone she should look at herself sitting and lying in front of a mirror, naked from the waist up. But if she does this she will see:

◆ how her breasts 'fall' when she is relaxed and her arms are down by her side
◆ where her areola and nipples are, and whether they point outwards, down to the floor, or out to the sides
◆ where her nipples and areolas are in relation to her forearms when her arms are folded across her body in as relaxed a way as possible; the shoulders and upper arms should not be brought forward (for this causes tension)
◆ how her breasts 'drape' on the bed or pillow, and where her nipples and areolas are when she lies on her side.

This information is invaluable. If the mother sees where her nipples and areolas are when she is sitting or lying down she has more understanding of how to position either her baby or herself for attachment. To do this she needs to know the following **key points of positioning**. These are:

1. The baby's nose or upper lip should be opposite the nipple.
2. The baby's head and body should be in a straight line.
3. The baby should be as close to the mother as possible.
4. If the baby is very small or newborn his bottom should also be supported.

The mother should not move her breasts from how they naturally fall. Positioning her baby should be adapted to take her breast shape,

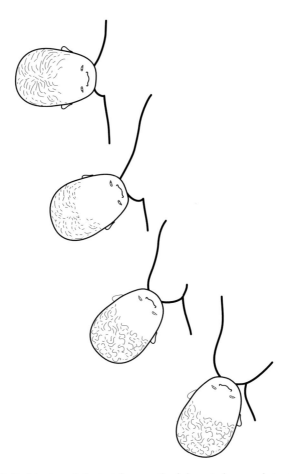

Figure 2.4 Positioning a baby to take a mother's breast shape and size into consideration.

size and position into consideration (Fig. 2.4). The one possible exception to this is if the mother has very large and heavy breasts which are also long. It can then be useful to support the breast in a sling made of soft material (a technique used by Chloe Fisher and Sally Inch in their breastfeeding clinic at the John Radcliffe Hospital, in Oxford). In hospital a wide piece of elasticated tubular bandage can be used. This is placed around the neck and down underneath the breast. It helps to make the nipple and areola complex more prominent and thus helps the baby to attach more easily. If this is used it is a good idea for the mother to observe her breast in a mirror to see how this changes the position of her nipples.

2.3 PRACTICAL POSITIONS FOR BREASTFEEDING

There are many positions in which a mother can breastfeed her baby. Initially, it is important that she finds a position in which she is comfortable and which is, therefore, most likely to lead to successful breastfeeding. Equally, it is essential for the mother to have her baby positioned in such a way that she is in control of helping him to attach to the breast herself and she is not dependent upon the help of a second person.

The mother may have definite views about which position she wishes to use (especially if she has breastfed before) and if these work for her that is fine. However, for a baby compromised by size or clinical condition, possible positions which may be more successful in the early days of feeding may be new to the mother, and it is important to explain why these different positions may be more appropriate until her baby is older and bigger.

It is useful to teach *all* mothers more than one position for breastfeeding. Different positions can be appropriate in a number of situations: for example, as small babies grow bigger and stronger; to give a mother flexibility if she is using an unconventional breastfeeding position at home (for any reason) but wishes to use a more conventional position when she goes out; and for babies before and after surgery, babies who have a cleft lip and palate, and so on. In addition, a baby's position at the breast may have direct influence on how effectively he is attached and, therefore, how efficiently he drains the whole breast, rather than only part of it. Hence, mothers who experience blocked lobes or mastitis may find that using another position for breastfeeding facilitates an improved attachment at the breast, thus achieving better drainage.

Positions for breastfeeding can be divided into three types: sitting, lying and leaning.

2.3.1 Sitting positions

The underarm position

The 'underarm' position is ideal for small and preterm babies, and for babies with poor head control. It is a useful position for newborn term babies too (Fig. 2.5). The advantages of this position are:

◆ When a baby has a small mouth, and the nipple and areola appear impossibly large, attachment is easier.
◆ It enables a mother to see the position of her baby's tongue, which needs to be in the floor of the mouth prior to attachment – rather than up in the roof of the mouth, which is often the case.
◆ It is a comfortable and secure way of holding a baby with one arm, leaving the mother's other arm free.

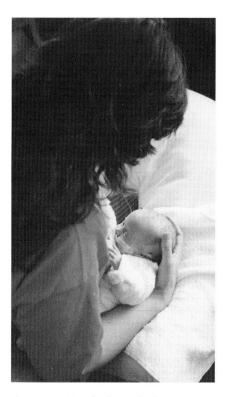

Figure 2.5 The underarm position for breastfeeding.

◆ The position can also be used at bath times, for washing the baby's hair.

How to position the baby using the underarm position

Initially, an easy way to teach the mother is to get her to stand up to position her baby. The baby should be held in a supine position with his lower body tucked into the mother's waist, just above her hip. The mother, using the arm on the same side of her body as the baby is positioned, supports the baby's head with her hand and uses the length of her forearm to support the full length of his body. When she then sits down her body is straight and she is more relaxed as a result. When the baby is positioned with the mother already sitting, she often unconsciously leans towards her baby and quickly becomes tired and uncomfortable. Once she has become accustomed to positioning her baby while standing up, she will be able to adopt the correct position for both herself and her baby more easily while sitting down.

To help the mother gain confidence in handling her baby, when she is standing up and has the baby positioned, encourage her to take him for a small walk around the area of the cot or incubator. Even if the baby is attached to an array of monitors, the mother can take a few steps with him in the underarm position. (If the baby is very fragile, it is best to postpone this walk until his condition is more stable.)

How to attach a baby in the underarm position to the breast

The mother should gently cup the baby's head in her hand, rather than grip the back of his head (Fig. 2.5), which may be painful and cause the baby to be irritable and pull away from the breast. Alternatively, the mother can support the base of her baby's head between her thumb and fingers (see Fig. 2.7). Supporting the baby's head gives the mother maximum control and enables her to slightly extend her baby's head, making it easier for him to suckle effectively. The mother may offer her baby the breast by positioning her four fingers under the breast and use her thumb and forefinger to shape the breast on either side of, but not too close to, the nipple and areola (using the same hand-hold as for hand expression). In this position it is easy to touch and lightly brush the baby's mouth or cheek with the nipple, to encourage the 'rooting' reflex, that is, the baby turning his head towards the breast with his mouth opened widely (Fig. 2.6). At this point the mother should move the baby quickly onto the breast, making sure the baby's upper lip or nose is opposite her nipple before attachment. Once the baby is correctly attached, the mother should take her fingers away from the breast.

The mother may need to use a towel or small blanket to help support her baby and her arm.

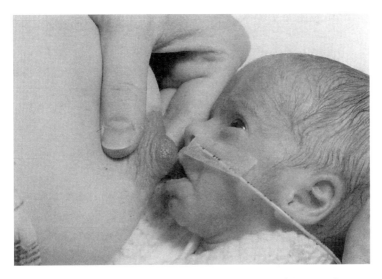

Figure 2.6 Encouraging a preterm baby to open his mouth (photograph courtesy of the North Staffs Neonatal Unit).

The traditional position

The traditional position is the most commonly seen breastfeeding position, in which the baby is held across the mother's chest. There are two main variations:

◆ The mother rests her baby's head on her forearm, supporting his shoulders and back with her hand; with a small baby she should also support his bottom. This is suitable for babies with good head control, for example most term, healthy babies (see Fig. 2.8).
◆ The mother supports the baby's head with the hand opposite the breast from which the baby is feeding (Fig. 2.7). This is suitable for small babies and for babies with poor head control.

How to hold a baby using the traditional position

When initially learning to hold a baby for this position it is a good idea to combine both variations. To start with, the mother supports her baby's head with her hand, giving her enough control to slightly extend his head which makes attachment easier to achieve. She must ensure her nipple is opposite either the baby's nose or upper lip – a mirror can be useful here. Once the baby has attached to the breast there is a choice:

◆ The mother can continue to support her baby's head with the same hand for the complete feed, making sure she has a towel or small

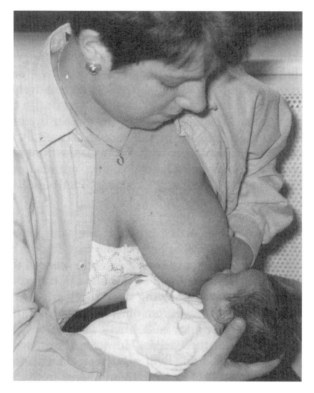

Figure 2.7 The 'traditional' position for breastfeeding (photograph courtesy of the North Staffs Neonatal Unit).

blanket to support either her baby or her hand or arm so that she can maintain the position.

◆ Alternatively, she can fold her other arm across her body at right angles (the arm on the same side as the breast from which the baby is feeding). She should gradually raise her arm till she can support the weight of her baby and take the hand supporting her baby's head away. This arm then supports her baby's back and bottom, particularly if the baby is newborn.

The mother should not move her breasts. She should always take her baby to the breast, not the other way round. If she has looked at herself in the mirror she may have observed where her nipples were in relation to her forearm – if she can remember where that was, it will be approximately where the baby's mouth should be. The baby should be held close to the mother with his legs tucked around her body.

A term baby who is able to breastfeed without difficulty may have no problem with his head resting on the mother's forearm, but for a small or weak baby it is beneficial if the mother supports her baby's head with her hand to maintain good attachment, particularly in the early days. Once the baby is older and stronger the baby will need less head support and the mother can use either of the two variations described.

If the mother's breasts point out to the sides and her nipples face towards the crook of the elbow it may be comfortable in the first few days for the baby to rest his head in the crook of her arm; but gradually as the baby's head and body grow she will have to move her elbow further out at an angle, which cannot easily be maintained without support.

As babies grow bigger it is important to remember that the back, shoulders and the bottom cannot be supported with only one hand and arm; both arms should be used.

A baby who appears to 'prefer' to feed from one breast more than the other, will often take both sides equally well if held by the mother using her 'preferred' arm, for both breasts. For example, the baby can breast-feed from the 'preferred' breast first of all, held in the traditional position, with his head supported in the mother's hand. To feed from the other side, the baby should be moved across to the other breast without turning him around. He will still be facing the same direction as for the first breast. He will now be in the underarm position, but is supported with the mother's same hand and arm as for the first breast. It makes no difference which breast the baby initially feeds from, as long as the mother either uses the traditional position for the first side, followed by the underarm position for the other breast; or she starts off using the underarm position for the first breast, and then uses the traditional position for the other side.

When using a traditional position beware of trying to hold the baby, as some books and leaflets suggest, 'chest to chest'. The baby needs to be held to face the breast he is feeding from, and particularly the nipple and areola he will take into his mouth. His head and body need to be kept in line opposite this part of the breast. It is commonly the case that holding a baby 'chest to chest' results in him turning his head away from his body, so that he can no longer maintain his attachment.

Other sitting positions

Sitting cross-legged either on the floor or on a bed provides a comfortable and stable position for breastfeeding. The mother's thighs provide a natural support for her arms when she is holding her baby (Fig. 2.8). She may need pillows or cushions behind her back.

In Chapter 6 two other sitting positions are described which can be used with babies with cleft palate abnormalities (see Figs 6.1 and 6.2).

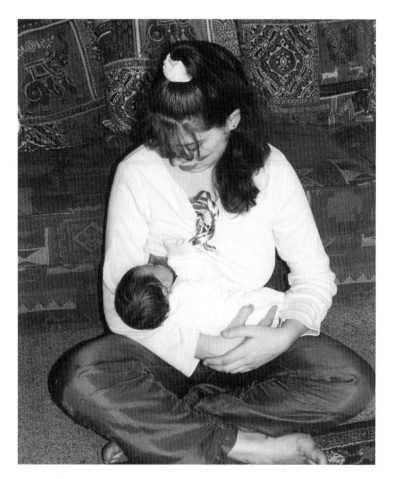

Figure 2.8 Sitting cross-legged.

A variation of the position shown in Fig. 6.2 is with the baby sitting astride the mother's thigh, rather than with both legs to one side. Both of these positions are useful for a baby suffering from gastro-oesophageal reflux, where having the baby in a sitting position can help reduce the incidence of vomiting. A baby wearing a Pavlik harness, or a plaster cast or double nappies to remedy congenital dislocation of the hip, may find the position illustrated in Fig. 6.2 helpful.

2.3.2 Lying-down positions

Some positions in which the mother lies down to breastfeed are very helpful to babies who need special care. There are two main positions

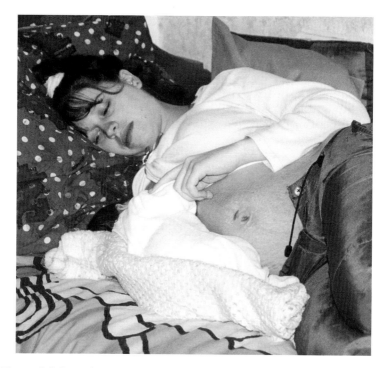

Figure 2.9 Lying down to breastfeed.

she can adopt:

◆ lying on her side with the baby alongside, either on his back or on his side (Fig. 2.9)
◆ lying on her back with the baby lying on her abdomen or across her chest.

Either of these positions is useful for:

◆ a mother who has had a caesarean section
◆ a mother who is disabled and cannot take the weight of the baby in her arms
◆ a mother who is unable for some reason to sit up
◆ a baby who has a cleft lip and/or palate
◆ a baby who has poor head control
◆ a baby who refuses to breastfeed when the mother holds him in sitting positions
◆ a weary mother! A lying position maximizes her chance to rest comfortably
◆ ensuring a mother can feed her baby at night in her bed.

How to help a mother lying down to breastfeed

The mother lying on her side

A mother needs at least two soft, comfortable pillows for her head. She may need another soft pillow to put under her waist or under her shoulders and chest. If she has large breasts a pillow under her shoulders and chest may elevate her sufficiently to prevent her breasts from 'flopping' on the bed and making it difficult for the baby to easily reach the nipple and areola.

◆ The breasts may need to be slightly over the edge of the pillow, which means about 5–10 cm of pillow is showing beyond the mother's chest wall. This ensures that sufficient nipple and surrounding breast tissue can be taken into the baby's mouth. A soft pillow, rather than one that is firm or hard, or a towel can be used under the mother, so that the nipple and areola are about the same level as the baby's mouth – but not higher (see Fig. 2.10).

◆ A soft pillow under the mother's chest, level with her chest wall, may be all that is required to elevate her enough for the baby to easily attach at the breast.

The mother may find an additional soft pillow or rolled-up towel or blanket put behind her back gives her support and helps her maintain her position. Whether the mother lies exactly on her side or slightly forward depends upon the size of her breasts. If her breasts are small, she may find it easier to feed just from the side on which she is lying, turning over to feed from the other breast. If her breasts are larger, the mother may find she can feed from the breast on the side on which she is lying, and then lean forward slightly to feed from the other breast, without the need to turn over.

It is important for the mother to make sure her arms are comfortably positioned. She may find having the arm on the side she is lying, stretched up and slightly forward under her pillow is comfortable. With her other arm she can support the back of her baby. The mother needs to experiment with different arm positions to find ones that are comfortable for her.

The baby can lie alongside the mother on his side and be supported along his back by a rolled-up small towel, or by the mother's arm and hand. If the mother has a blocked lobe or mastitis it may be beneficial if her baby lies alongside his mother, with his feet towards the head of the bed instead of towards the foot of the bed (Fig. 2.10).

The baby can lie flat on his back as in Fig. 6.3 with the mother positioned so that she is leaning forward over her baby with her breast falling into his mouth. This is a useful position for any mother who feels very anxious about holding her baby in her arms to breastfeed. It works

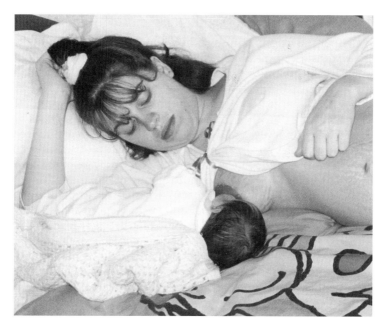

Figure 2.10 A baby lying with his feet towards the head of the bed.

well as long as the baby has sufficient breast tissue in his mouth. The mother should try not to sleep like this, as it is not a stable position.

The mother lying on her back

A mother can lie on her back to breastfeed. She may find it more comfortable not to be completely flat, but to have two or three pillows under her head and shoulders and a pillow under her upper back. The baby can be arranged in a number of positions:

◆ The baby can lie on the mother's abdomen towards one of her breasts so that he can easily reach the nipple and areola. In this position the mother may have to lightly support his forehead when he feeds, as in Fig. 5.1. The mother may find it comfortable to bend her knees and rest her feet flat on the bed. She can support her baby with her arms.

◆ If the mother is lying flat on her back, the baby can be placed over her shoulder with his legs resting on a pillow. In this way the baby can effectively drain lobes of the breast that are more prone to blockage.

◆ A baby with his legs in a plaster cast or Pavlik harness (for congenital dislocation of the hips) can be placed on a pillow by the side of the mother, and laid across her chest so that he can reach her nipple and areola.

The mother may need assistance with these positions.

Should a mother and her baby sleep together?

Throughout the world mothers, fathers and babies sleep together, and enjoy what is a very pleasurable and special time. This has been happening for millennia. A number of studies have shown that 'bed-sharing' helps to establish and promote breastfeeding.[4] In one report the number of times the baby fed was greater during the night, compared with babies who slept on their own.[5] Night feeding helps to boost the mother's prolactin levels and increases her milk production. Moreover, mothers and babies appear to be very aware of each other when they sleep together.[6] Unfortunately, we also have to be aware of the recommendations from the Foundation for the Study of Infant Deaths, which says that mothers should 'put the baby back in its cot to sleep'.[7] Parents will be confused by this apparently contradictory information.

If a mother would like to sleep throughout the night with her baby, whether she is at home or in hospital, or is advised to spend the day in bed with her baby, there are a number of important points she should consider. A baby should **not** sleep in the same bed as his mother and father if either of them smoke, regularly drink alcohol, or take drugs that make them sleepy, or recreational drugs such as cannabis. In these cases, after breastfeeding, the baby should **always** be returned to his own cot. Smoking has been shown to increase the risk of sudden infant death syndrome, and alcohol and drug-taking may make the mother and/or her partner sleep very heavily and possibly roll over on top of their baby. If possible, smoking should be done outside the house not inside, and certainly not in the room in which the baby sleeps.

There will, however, always be times when a mother snoozes or sleeps while feeding her baby. If the baby is taken into his parents' or mother's bed during the night, then there will be occasions when all fall asleep together. As long as the above situations do not apply, these times should be treasured.[8] To say to a mother 'you must not sleep with your baby' is unrealistic, as it is known that babies commonly spend part of the night in their parents bed.[9] So! The advice to give to mothers needs to be how to ensure the safety of the baby and look at the risk factors he is being exposed to – and the benefits, particularly with respect to the establishment of breastfeeding and its duration.

If the baby regularly comes into his parents' bed, it is better for blankets to be used rather than duvets. Duvets may be too hot; babies do not regulate their temperatures particularly well and they can easily get too warm. If a duvet is used the baby should be placed on the top of the duvet, on his back, and covered with his normal covers.

If the mother is likely to sleep while feeding it is important for her to feed in a position in which she is 'stable'; in other words, where she cannot roll over onto her baby, if she goes to sleep. To stop herself rolling she needs to bend her legs and draw them up to her body, and then straighten out her top leg. A pillow between her legs will increase her comfort. She will find this a comfortable position, which allows her to curl herself around her baby, but without being able to roll onto him. If the bed is against a wall make sure there is no gap between the bed and the wall for him to fall between. It is better not to put the baby where he is in danger of falling off the bed. It is better not to feed him lying on a sofa; he may get trapped in the area between the seat and the back.

Strongly encourage the mother to have her baby sleep in the same room as herself. Put the cot next to her bed – so that even if the baby does not sleep with his parents, the mother can still touch him easily, and he is close by for night feeds. If a mother can come into hospital to stay for one or more nights before her baby is discharged this is an ideal opportunity for her to become used to her baby being in the same room and perhaps in the same bed.

2.3.3 Less conventional and leaning positions

There are a number of less conventional breastfeeding positions, which enable a mother to successfully breastfeed for a short time until a more conventional position can be used.

◆ A modification of the underarm position is useful if a baby needs to be fed while lying flat. This may arise if the baby is wearing a plaster splint or has had abdominal surgery, or has an oral defect such as a cleft lip and palate (unilateral or bilateral), where it may be an advantage if the areola and nipple fall directly into the baby's mouth. The baby may be in a cot with sides that can be removed, or on a bed or on a chair. He should be positioned so that he can remain flat with his lower body and legs supported on a pillow so that he is level with his mother's lap. The mother does not need to support his body with her forearm, but she should support his head in her hand. The baby should be in a position where she can easily lean forward and let her breast fall into his mouth. She may require a second person to help adjust the position of the baby so that his whole body is aligned. She should make sure she is comfortable

◆ The mother may find it helps to have a table in front of her with a comfortable pillow to lean her head on so that her back does not become tired or stiff. The advantage of this position is that she has one hand free to help with attachment or to express milk directly into her baby's mouth.

◆ The baby can be laid flat on the floor, on a table or on a chair. His head should be towards the mother with his feet facing away from her. The mother can lean across the baby so that her breast falls into her baby's mouth (Fig. 2.11). Most mothers find they can support themselves by leaning on their elbows. One mother was observed reading a

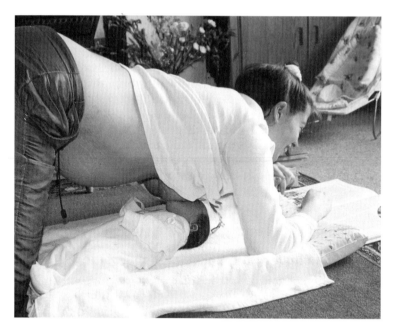

Figure 2.11 A mother leaning across her baby to feed.

book in a cookery-book stand while feeding a baby in this position! She had inverted nipples and found this position worked during the day for the first two weeks after birth. At night she slept with her baby and let her breast fall into his mouth whenever he wanted to feed.

◆ A mother with 'too much' milk, which flows very quickly, may find reclining in a chair or lying in a semi-reclining position on a bed slows the milk flow sufficiently for her baby to feed comfortably. Lying on her back can be helpful in slowing the milk flow too.

◆ A mother can breastfeed while standing or sitting upright if she has a sling around her shoulder and around her baby's bottom on the opposite side. The baby is sitting very upright facing the breast. She supports the baby's head and shoulders with her hand.

2.3.4 Breastfeeding more than one baby at each feed

Mothers feeding more than one baby at the same time can use a combination of positions. Twins, for example, can be held with both in the underarm positions – one on each side, or both in the traditional position. Alternatively, one twin can be held in the traditional position and one in the underarm position. Whichever position the mother is most comfortable in and can manage herself should be used. A V-shaped pillow placed around her with the V at the front may help in supporting twins. These positions are also suitable for mothers who are tandem feeding, i.e. feeding a newborn baby and an older child at the same time.

The mother may experience initial difficulties with positioning two babies at the breast at the same time and finding a comfortable position herself. To begin with it may be easier to position her babies and even feed them separately. Once they are fed and settled she can experiment with different ways of holding them together.

Twins commonly feed from only one breast each. This is not normally a problem, for each breast is quite able to provide sufficient milk for their needs. However, if one twin is bigger than the other, or if one twin gains weight more quickly than the other, it may help to swap them to feed from the opposite breast (i.e. the breast they do not usually feed from). In this way the breasts are both stimulated to produce adequate amounts of milk.

2.3.5 Positioning, monitoring and oxygen therapy

Many of the babies in a neonatal or specialist paediatric unit are likely to require some form of monitoring – measuring heart rate, respiration or oxygen saturation. In most cases this involves a cable between the monitoring apparatus and the baby. Breastfeeding a baby attached to a large monitor should not be a problem as long as the mother's chair is close enough to the monitor to ensure that all connections are secure.

Small portable monitors, measuring respirations, can easily be tucked into the blanket or sheet used to wrap the baby, or else they can simply be placed in the mother's lap. Often the small respiration monitors can be disconnected while the mother is holding her baby.

A baby receiving oxygen should also have no problems breastfeeding, as long as the oxygen requirement is not so high as to necessitate the baby receiving it via a headbox. A funnel placed over the mother's shoulder, near the baby's face, should be adequate if he does not have nasal cannulae. As with monitor cables, it is important to be sure the mother's chair is close enough to the source of oxygen and that any tubes are long enough, without being pulled taut when the mother and baby are comfortably positioned in a chair.

2.4 BREAST ATTACHMENT

'Attachment' is the ability of the baby to take a generous amount of breast tissue into his mouth so that when he suckles, milk is effectively removed from the lactiferous sinuses.

Successful breastfeeding depends upon the baby being able to repeatedly drain the lactiferous sinuses. To do this the baby must take

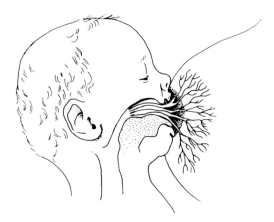

Figure 2.12 An inside view of the breast when attachment is good.

much of the areola into his mouth, forming a long 'teat' from the breast tissue,[1] with the nipple forming approximately one-third of this teat. The baby's tongue is to the front of his mouth and positioned over his lower gums, beneath the lactiferous sinuses. It is 'cupped' round the 'teat' of breast tissue. The tongue moves in a wave-like action from the front to the back. This 'wave' causes the 'teat' of breast tissue to be pressed against the hard palate, which squeezes the milk out of the lactiferous sinuses into the baby's mouth (Fig. 2.12).

The baby does not 'suck' the milk out of the breast. Suction helps to form the long 'teat' and then holds the breast tissue in the baby's mouth. The milk is removed by rhythmic compression and release of the lactiferous sinuses. The breast tissue does not move once inside the baby's mouth, therefore if attachment is correct there should be no damage to the nipple or breast tissue. Neither should breastfeeding be painful, though some mothers may experience discomfort initially until they are used to the sensation.

To attach a baby correctly

The **key points** are:

1. The baby's head and body should be in a straight line.
2. His head and body should face the breast, with his nose or upper lip opposite his mother's nipple.
3. His mouth should be widely open (this can be encouraged by touching the baby's cheek or lips with a finger or nipple).
4. When he opens his mouth widely he needs to be moved quickly onto the breast.

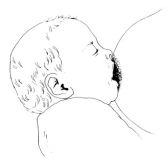

Figure 2.13 An outside view of the breast when attachment is good.

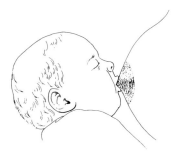

Figure 2.14 An outside view of the breast when attachment is poor.

5. The baby's lower lip should be aimed below the mother's nipple so that his chin touches the breast. A possible exception to this may be when positioning and attaching a baby with a small lower jaw, such as in Pierre Robin syndrome; then the baby's chin should be as close to the mother's breast as possible.
6. More of the mother's areola should be visible above the baby's mouth than below it (Fig. 2.13).

If the mother aims her nipple and areola towards the centre of the mouth, the nipple soon comes into contact with the tongue and cannot go far enough back into the mouth. In this case the baby appears to be nipple sucking only even though his mouth was widely open when he attached to the breast.

Signs of poor attachment

If the baby is poorly attached (Fig. 2.14) **the following signs are likely to be seen:**[1]

◆ The baby's chin does not touch the mother's breast.

- The baby's mouth is not widely open and his lips may almost be closed.
- The baby's lower lip is not turned outwards, instead his lips are pursed forwards.
- The same amount of areola can be seen above and below the baby's mouth. This indicates that the mother's nipple was aimed centrally into the baby's mouth (a very common mistake).

Results of poor attachment

The results of poor attachment include:

- breast engorgement
- sore or cracked nipples
- an unsettled baby because the milk is not flowing quickly enough
- a baby who wants to feed very often or for long periods
- a baby who refuses to feed, gains weight very slowly or who begins to lose weight.

2.4.1 How to remove a baby from the breast

If for any reason a mother needs to take her baby off the breast before a feed is finished, or because the baby has not attached to the breast comfortably, the easiest and most effective way is for the mother to insert her little finger into the side of the baby's mouth to break the seal around the breast tissue, and then gently remove him from the breast.

Sore or damaged nipples and areola can result from pulling the baby from the breast before the seal around the breast tissue has been broken.

2.4.2 How to help a baby with difficulty attaching to the breast

Some babies have difficulty becoming attached to the breast because they have very low energy levels, or have a specific weakness of the muscles involved in feeding caused by a neurological or chromosomal abnormality. If this weakness affects their lower jaw, the following hand position may be useful.

The mother supporting both her breast and her baby's chin at the same time enhances the baby's attachment at the breast. In this way, the mother is able to assist the baby to maintain his attachment, so that when he pauses or becomes tired his lower jaw does not fall away from the breast and affect his attachment. This position for attachment is known as the 'Dancer' position (Fig. 2.15). To use this technique, the mother should:

1. Position the baby comfortably at the breast in an upright sitting position.

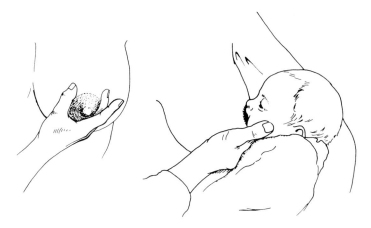

Figure 2.15 The Dancer position for attachment at the breast.

2. Make sure the baby is well supported (use small blankets or towels if necessary) and the hand opposite the breast is free.
3. Place her thumb and first finger on either side of the baby's chin.
4. Support the breast with the palm of her hand and the other three fingers.
5. When the baby opens his mouth and is attached to the breast, continue to support his head and chin as described.

2.4.3 How to attach a baby to the breast who has become used to a bottle teat or dummy

Both a dummy and the teat of a bottle provide a hard, unyielding and constant stimulus to the area between the hard and soft palate. This stimulates the baby to suck. If the baby becomes used to this stimuli, attachment at the breast may be more difficult. This is because the nipple and areola of the breast are softer and produce a more subtle form of palate stimulation. However, it may be useful if a mother gently massages the nipple for a few seconds just before attachment, so that it becomes hard or more erect, and then follows the steps to attachment given in section 2.4.2. Slight pressure from the mother's forefinger or thumb on the top of the areola (approximately 2.5 cm from the nipple) usually results in the nipple facing slightly upwards. If this is done at the time of attachment it may help the 'hardened' nipple to come into contact with the palate and thus initiate a sucking response.

Babies who may benefit from this help include:

◆ preterm babies who have been given dummies for comfort over a long period, particularly if they refuse the breast

◆ preterm babies who have been given bottles before they are established at the breast; these babies may also initially refuse to breastfeed
◆ term babies who have been given bottles or dummies, and who refuse to breastfeed because they may have developed a preference for the stimulation provided by a teat.

2.5 HOW LONG SHOULD A FEED LAST?

Clocks have no place in timing feeds for term, healthy babies. If a baby is in the correct position and suckling properly, the feed should last until the baby is satisfied and comes off the breast himself. No two babies will feed for the same length of time. A term baby should have as long as he wants on the first breast and should then be offered the other breast, which may or may not be taken. At each feed, the baby should be given alternate breasts so that each breast is equally stimulated. Some mothers find it helps them to remember which breast to start the feed from if they attach a safety pin or brooch on the appropriate side of their clothing.

In the case of preterm babies, and particularly those of 35 weeks or less and ill babies, it is equally important not to restrict the time they spend suckling at the breast. It is quite satisfactory not to offer the other breast if the baby is satisfied. As with the term, healthy baby, alternate breasts should be offered to the baby at each feed (although it may, in this case, be necessary to express the milk from the other side if the baby is not yet taking all the milk he requires from the breast).

While no time limit should be placed on a breastfeed, there are situations, particularly with babies less than 34 or 35 weeks, or those who have cardiac or respiratory problems, where feeds are obviously taking too long. One-and-a-half hours, for example, would not be normal for the majority of babies.

Poor or static weight gain is often associated with prolonged feeding times and is a further indication that a problem exists. If the breastfeeds are taking a very long time, there are a number of possible reasons:

◆ Poor positioning and attachment of the baby at the breast.
◆ A poor maternal milk supply, owing to a lack of effective stimulation.
◆ The baby has an immature or weak pattern of sucking, and is not able to drain the lactiferous sinuses or breast effectively.
◆ The baby has a clinical condition, making him sleepy or weak.

2.5.1 Remedies to use when feeding times are prolonged

◆ Ensure the baby is in an appropriate position for feeding according to his size and gestation. Check the baby is attached to the breast and not sucking only on the nipple. Teach the mother to support her baby's head with one hand so that when he opens his mouth widely she can use her other hand to guide her nipple and areola into his mouth, taking her hand away once attachment is achieved.

◆ If the baby has a weak, immature or uncoordinated suckling action, appropriate sucking practice may help – ideally this should be at the breast. A clean index or little finger may help you diagnose whether there is any uncoordinated tongue movement. Gently agitate the area between the baby's hard and soft palate with the pad of the finger. This should stimulate a sucking response. The finger should not be so far back in the baby's mouth that he gags. The tongue should move in a rhythmic way from the front to the back. Allow the baby to suck on your knuckle if possible for about half a minute before a feed.

◆ Examine the mother's present routine, particularly if she has recently gone home from hospital. She may be trying to get back into a 'normal' routine, thus reducing the regularity or length of expression or breastfeeding sessions. She may not be eating or drinking regularly if she has to visit her baby in a neonatal unit or has other children to care for. She may feel she has to do all the things she did before her baby also needed her, and may need help and support to recognize that her priorities are now likely to be different – and that one of her important priorities is to care for herself. She also needs to accept that life is unlikely to return to how it was before her baby was born.

◆ A mother of a baby with low energy reserves may find it beneficial to learn how to hand-express, so that she can use direct expression to start a breastfeed. If the mother has a good milk supply she should express a small quantity of milk prior to feeding, so that her baby obtains the fat-rich hind-milk more quickly. The milk already expressed may be given to the baby in a cup after the breastfeed, as this will require less energy expenditure. This regimen aims at increasing the baby's weight without him becoming too tired to feed orally.

◆ A jaundiced baby may be too sleepy to feed, in which case it will be counterproductive to try to wake him. It may be better to wait until he wakes naturally or, if there is any concern that the baby's condition will worsen as a result, to give him a feed by gastric tube.

2.6 HOW OFTEN SHOULD A BABY FEED?

Babies born at term who are healthy and for whom there is no medical contraindication should feed whenever they are hungry or thirsty, that is, 'on demand' or 'on request'. No time intervals should be imposed. This may mean that some babies sleep for long periods between breastfeeds in the first few days after birth. Thereafter, the frequency of feeding between individual babies may vary enormously. Some babies may feed as often as 10–12 times in 24 hours, while others may only feed five or six times. Both are normal. It is worth remembering that a baby's stomach at birth is not much bigger than a walnut. In a neonatal or paediatric unit, feeding regimens are rarely 'normal'; they exist to enable a set quantity of fluid to be given to a baby over a 24-hour period – left alone, a baby may have other ideas of how often he wishes to feed. Very occasionally the two may be the same!

There is evidence to suggest that babies who are unrestricted in frequency of feeds gain weight more rapidly.[10] On a neonatal unit a 3-hourly or 4-hourly feeding schedule may be considered necessary for some breastfed babies because of an existing clinical condition such as jaundice, although if a baby has to be woken, he will be less inclined to feed properly and take the full amounts. It is better to let the baby regulate himself as soon as possible.

If the baby is being tube-fed overnight, it is important to make sure the feeds are given regularly (3-hourly), so that more flexibility of timing feeds is possible during the day when the mother is available to feed. Daily or alternate-day weighing is an appropriate way of assessing the baby's progress and detecting any feeding problems.

Many babies do eventually establish a pattern of six to eight feeds in 24 hours, with more frequent feeds often required towards the evening. Night feeds are very important and mothers should not be encouraged to miss them while in hospital; otherwise, once the mother returns home with her baby, she may be totally unprepared for her baby's normal feeding pattern. Night feeds also help maintain her milk supply, particularly in the early days, by stimulating the production of prolactin.

During periods of rapid growth, which will occur in the first 2–3 months following delivery, a baby may want extra feeds. This often coincides with the time that many mothers give up breastfeeding, because they mistakenly believe their milk supply is no longer sufficient for the baby, who has suddenly become rather irritable and appears unsatisfied with his usual feeding regimen. This unsettled period lasts for 24–48 hours while the mother's milk supply adjusts to her baby's new needs. The routine then usually returns to the 'normal' feeding pattern for that baby.

Term babies who are having antibiotic therapy but who are otherwise well should be fed on demand. For term babies who are unwell, but are waking and requiring feeds, demand feeding is also suitable as they may require extra fluids and energy. A formal time schedule may interfere with this by restricting their fluid intake. Most jaundiced term babies will also be able to regulate their own feeding requirements.

2.6.1 The preterm baby

Babies of 36 weeks' gestation or less, and who are exclusively breast-feeding or having tube or cup feeds overnight, should be allowed to go 3–4 hours between feeds, as long as this is not medically contraindicated. Alternate daily weighing is recommended for this group of babies if fed on demand.

Preterm babies may initially require continuous pump feeds, until they are able to tolerate bolus feeds at hourly, 2-hourly or 3-hourly intervals. Once they can tolerate 2-hourly bolus feeds it is a mistake to believe that they will all eventually tolerate 3-hourly feeds. While it is common for 3-hourly or even 4-hourly feeds to be introduced during the time the baby is on a neonatal unit, it is essential for a mother to be aware that, when the baby goes home, he may feed according to his own individual needs – and these may be more frequent feeds: 10 or more breastfeeds in 24 hours is not unusual, and a 2-hourly feeding pattern during the day is very common. These babies have tiny stomachs! It is not a sign that the mother has an insufficient milk supply; it is just that baby's own personal feeding pattern. Many babies born at term and preterm will eventually develop a 3-hourly to 4-hourly feeding pattern, but this should not be expected. Such a feeding pattern is more common among formula-fed babies because gastric emptying times are longer and more consistent. This reflects the unchanging nature of formula milk. Human milk has a faster gastric emptying time because the nutrients are more easily absorbed by the baby; this is advantageous to the preterm baby.

2.7 HAS THE BABY HAD ENOUGH?

A baby who settles well between feeds, has around six wet nappies per day or more and is putting on weight is getting sufficient milk. It is usual for babies to lose some weight in the first week of life. By day 10–14, most healthy, term babies will have regained their birthweight. This will not apply if a baby is very preterm or very poorly – it may then take longer for the baby to regain his birthweight. How much longer will depend on the individual circumstances of the baby.

During the first 7–10 days, while the mother is still experiencing the feeling of breast fullness prior to feeding, it is useful to encourage her to gently handle her breasts, to get to know how they feel before and after a feed. This will give her the confidence to know that her baby has had sufficient milk. She can be assured that if her breasts are soft and comfortable following a feed, then her baby is getting sufficient milk – particularly if the points in the paragraph above are taken into consideration.

2.8 THE BABY'S NEED FOR ORAL STIMULATION AND NON-NUTRITIVE SUCKING

In utero babies have practice and experience of sucking and swallowing so that, when born at term, most are capable of breastfeeding within a very short time of birth.

For the preterm baby, depending upon his gestation at birth, this opportunity to 'prime' the structures involved in feeding is incomplete. However, many preterm babies show a desire for oral stimulation of some kind. It is particularly noticeable, for example, in some preterm babies that they open and close their mouths and protrude their tongue during intermittent gastric tube feeds. This may be due to subtle temperature changes experienced by the baby during the feed.

Some preterm babies who are ventilated for any length of time may have considerable oral stimulation from the endotracheal tube. As a consequence, some are able to suckle quite well after extubation (even a baby as young as 28 weeks post-conception age who is held close to the mother's breast after extubation may lick any milk expressed on to the nipple, and some may attempt to suckle). This appears to be a temporary skill, however, which disappears quite quickly, only to reappear when the baby is more mature and developmentally more able to coordinate his skills safely.

What kind of oral stimulation should be given to a baby who is preterm, ill, or has an oral defect? For the preterm baby there is a need to provide some form of developmentally appropriate stimulation, which at the same time provides comfort to the baby. For the full-term, ill baby the need for comfort may be acute, and for the baby with an oral defect or a neurological condition it may be important to provide stimulation to the palate and tongue to encourage correct feeding movements. The kind of oral stimulation a baby receives, particularly if he is in a neonatal or paediatric unit, may be extensive. It may range from being very unpleasant, though necessary or even life-saving – for example, oral intubation, oral suctioning, the making and fitting of a dental plate (or obturator), the passing of oral gastric feeding tubes, perhaps even mouth care – to being a positive and pleasurable stimulation, such as licking milk from the nipple or suckling at the breast. It may include sucking on a dummy, a bottle teat, a nipple shield, a finger or the baby's own fist, taking milk from a cup, or from the tube of a nursing supplementer.

What has to be considered for each individual baby is the kind of oral stimulation that is absolutely necessary, what is preferable as far as the establishment of breastfeeding is concerned, and what should be avoided if possible. A point of conflict in assessing the needs of a baby who is to breastfeed is how to provide oral stimulation that can comfort him if his mother is not present, or that can calm him when, for example, he exhibits signs of wanting something in his mouth at the time of being fed by gastric tube.

It is important to distinguish the baby's possible need for oral 'gratification', which may require some form of oral stimulation, and his need to be comforted. For a baby who is to be breastfed, both needs can be provided by the mother. Therefore, it is important for her to introduce her baby to the breast as early as possible. A baby will derive a lot of comfort from suckling as well as satisfying his oral and nutritive needs. Whether the baby is sick or preterm, comfort can be provided in a number of ways – even when the mother is not present. Sometimes it is tempting to give a baby a dummy when what the baby really wants is to be held and spoken to or caressed. A mother or a health professional can carry a baby in a sling. Sometimes all that is required is a tape recording of his parents' voices or gentle music or sounds, or even a breast pad or piece of clothing with his mother's familiar breast scent (in the same way as an article of the baby's clothing can provide comfort to the mother).

If the baby is obviously looking for some sort of oral stimulation and his mother is not present, it may be appropriate to give him a cup feed (rather than a gastric tube feed and a dummy). A cup feed will stimulate his tongue, lingual lipases, and his oral and nasal sensory receptors, without expecting him to have anything in his mouth, which he may find difficult to control, particularly if he is still very immature (30–32 weeks' gestation, for example). A cup feed may be especially appropriate for a baby with an oral defect or a neurological condition, who needs to strengthen his oral musculature and encourage a rhythmic tongue movement.

The tongue is an important sensory organ capable of providing pleasurable experiences. It is therefore important to use it to help a baby who has been subjected to any of the unpleasant oral stimuli previously mentioned. Cup-feeding makes use of the tongue: it encourages its movement in order to obtain the milk from the cup. All that is in the mouth is the milk coating the tongue (preferably the mother's breastmilk), so there is little chance of the baby having an unpleasant experience or panicking. Furthermore, cup-feeding provides a 'self-regulated' oral experience. If the baby is stimulated he takes milk; if he is not, he takes none. It is useful to provide a baby with an oral feeding experience that will not interfere with breastfeeding, but at the same time will satisfy his need for oral stimulation and require the person giving the feed to talk to and to hold the baby.

When a baby breastfeeds, a similar 'self-regulation' process occurs, for it is the baby who decides on the pace of the feed, when to begin and when to finish suckling. For a preterm baby who still has to learn to breastfeed, the best oral stimulation is provided at his mother's breast. Skin-to-skin contact is beneficial for it gives the baby ready access to the breast. The mother can express a little milk on to her nipples, or express directly into her baby's mouth, and she can help him attach to the breast. If he is ill, with very little energy, or still very young (32–35 weeks' gestation), he may be content simply to hold the breast tissue in his mouth. Suckling may not occur until he is ready, which may not be for several days or even weeks. The baby will decide when he is ready for another kind of oral stimulation and often this will be dictated by his own individual developmental 'clock'. The significance of this is not to force an immature baby to do anything he is not yet ready to do. Orally, this means avoiding the use of bottles until a baby is able to cope with them. As the skill of cup-feeding, appears to precede efficient breast-feeding, and breastfeeding appears to be possible before bottle-feeding, it may be prudent to avoid bottles altogether or at least until the baby and his mother have breastfeeding well established.

Oral stimulation can enhance or detract from the establishment of breastfeeding.[11,12] Dummies are often used in neonatal and paediatric units, but they are not pliable like the breast. They are static in the mouth and do not encourage the same movements of the tongue, lips or oral muscles as required in suckling. This is also true of the bottle teat, nipple shield and a finger. Nevertheless, there may be times when any one of these forms of oral stimulation is used (the bottle and dummy preferably with the permission of the parents). Where possible their use should be minimized so that the predominant oral stimulation experienced by a baby is at his mother's breast.

2.8.1 Non-nutritive sucking

Non-nutritive sucking describes the kind of sucking a baby might do without deriving any nutritive value from the activity. This can occur at the breast or on an inanimate object such as a dummy or a finger. Non-nutritive sucking may be used to calm a distressed baby, or when a procedure is about to take place, the unpleasant effect of which may be minimized by the baby sucking. The advantages of this occurring at the breast are the comforting effects of hearing his mother's heart beat, and the reassurance of being close to her with, her familiar smell and touch. Non-nutritive sucking is usually very fast, with two and a half sucking sequences per second, which is approximately twice the rate of nutritive sucking. Each sucking burst lasts around 3–4 seconds, with rests of 3–10 seconds in between.[13]

Among the reported benefits of non-nutritive sucking are an increased duration of breastfeeding. This has been associated with non-nutritive sucking at the breast when it is 'emptied'.[14] This is a technique that can be used to help increase the mother's milk production if it has begun to decrease – and to avoid the use of dummies. The mother puts her baby to the breast *after* she has expressed her milk. Non-nutritive sucking may also influence rates of growth in preterm babies, although this has still not been conclusively proved.[15]

Some preterm babies have also been observed to have increased transcutaneous oxygen levels during non-nutritive sucking.

REFERENCES

1. WHO/UNICEF (1993) *Breastfeeding Counselling: A Training Course.* Secretariat, Division of Diarrhoeal and Acute Respiratory Disease Control, Session 3, pp. 39–54. WHO, Geneva.
2. Nyqvist KH, Sjoden PO, Ewald U (1999) The development of preterm infants' breastfeeding behaviour. *Early Hum Dev* **55**: 247–264.
3. Hurst NM, Valentine CJ, Renfro L et al (1997) Skin-to-skin holding in the neonatal intensive care unit influences maternal milk volume. *J. Perinatol* **17**: 213–217.
4. Mosko S, McKenna J, Dickel M et al (1993) Parent-infant co-sleeping: the appropriate context for the study of infant sleep and implications for sudden infant death syndrome (SIDS) research. *J. Behav Med* **16**: 589–610.
5. McKenna J, Mosko S, Richard et al (1994) Experimental studies of infant–parent co-sleeping: mutual physiological and behavioural influences and their relevance to SIDS (sudden infant death syndrome). *Early Hum Dev* **38**: 187–201.
6. McKenna JJ, Mosko S, Richard CA (1997) Bedsharing promotes breastfeeding. *Pediatrics* **100**: 214–219.
7. Foundation for the Study of Infant Deaths (1997) *Questions and Answers about Cot Death.* London: FSID.
8. Jackson D (1990) *Three in a Bed: Why you Should Sleep with Your Baby.* London: Bloomsbury.
9. Ball H, Hooker E, Kelly P (1999) Where will the baby sleep? Attitudes and practices of new and experienced parents regarding cosleeping with their newborn infants. *Am. Anthropol* **101**: 143–150.
10. Illingworth RS, Stone DG (1952) Self-demand feeding in a maternity unit. *Lancet* i: 683–687.
11. Victora CG, Tomasi E, Olinto MTA et al (1993) Use of pacifiers and breastfeeding duration. *Lancet* **341**: 401–406.
12. Righard L, Alade MO (1992) Sucking technique and its effect on success of breastfeeding. *Birth* **19**: 185–189.
13. Coulter McBride M, Coulter Danner S (1987) Sucking disorders in neurologically impaired infants: assessment and facilitation of breastfeeding. *Clin Perinatol* **14**: 109–130.
14. Narayan I, Mehta R, Choudhury DK et al (1991) Sucking on the 'emptied breast': non-nutritive sucking with a difference. *Arch Dis Child* **66**: 241–244.
15. Bernbaum JC, Pereira GR, Watkins JB et al (1983) Non-nutritive sucking during gavage feeding enhances growth and maturation in preterm babies. *Pediatrics* **71**: 41–45.

The expression of breastmilk

3.1 HAND-EXPRESSION

The expression of breastmilk by hand is a skill that all mothers who are going to breastfeed should have the opportunity to learn. The reasons for teaching a mother to hand-express are:

- to ensure she is able to handle her breasts correctly without damaging the delicate breast tissue
- to help her to know how her breasts feel before and after a feed – giving a mother confidence about how much milk her baby has taken at each breastfeed
- to give a mother confidence that her body is working normally: she may feel that her body has failed her, if she has given birth to a preterm or sick baby
- to give her control over her own body and its milk production
- to enable a mother to express sufficient milk for a feed if her baby cannot be breastfed, either immediately after birth or on a later occasion; for example, if the mother returns to work, or if she or her baby becomes ill
- to enable a mother to express milk straight into her baby's mouth; this is useful when the baby is preterm and just beginning to learn to feed, because it stimulates his digestive juices (including the lingual lipases), and encourages the movement of his tongue and jaw muscles
- to help a baby to attach at the breast by the expression of a little milk onto the mother's nipple; this is particularly helpful for the preterm baby when he is learning to feed, or for a baby who tires quickly, and may also be useful for babies with Down's syndrome or a cleft lip and/or palate
- to enable the expression of some fore-milk if the mother has an abundant milk supply and the baby is unable to obtain the fat-rich

hind-milk because he has low energy reserves and cannot yet complete a feed
◆ to express a little milk prior to a feed to soften the mother's nipples, if they have become flattened due to engorgement or breast fullness; this will help a baby to attach to the breast correctly
◆ to express any lobes of the breast that become blocked – it is, therefore, one of the 'first-aid' measures in preventing mastitis (it may be used in conjunction with massage, see section 3.8.2.)
◆ to gently smooth a small amount of hind-milk over the nipple area after a feed or expression to help prevent the delicate skin from becoming too dry
◆ to help her relax: some mothers find hand-expression more acceptable than using a mechanical pump
◆ to reduce the risk of contamination: milk expressed by pump has a higher level of bacterial contamination
◆ to enable small amounts of colostrum to be collected more efficiently than by pump
◆ to produce milk with a higher sodium content and concentration than pump-expressed milk,[1] this may be advantageous to preterm babies of less than 30 weeks' gestation, who may have excessive sodium loss due to immature renal function.[2]

3.1.1 When and how often to hand-express

If a baby cannot breastfeed after birth, for whatever reason, the expression of milk by hand or mechanical pump is necessary. This should be commenced on the day of birth (if possible). The colostrum produced in these first days is vital for all babies, and particularly for those born preterm or who are ill. Therefore, if breastfeeding cannot begin within a few hours of birth, breastmilk should be expressed:

◆ as soon as possible after birth, within the first 6 hours if possible
◆ at least six to eight times in a 24-hour period – i.e. every 2–3 hours during the day, sometimes more
◆ at least once during the night
◆ with no time limits set, because the length of expression will vary with each mother
◆ as often as her baby would have breastfed
◆ for approximately a total of 20 minutes at each expression, or for more than 100 minutes in 24 hours.[3]

Practically, it is much easier to teach a mother the principles of hand-expression when her breasts are soft. If she does not begin expression until day 2 or 3, she is less likely to learn the skill easily, because it may be more uncomfortable and even painful to learn when there is venous engorgement and her breasts are full of milk. There is good evidence to suggest that the earlier a mother begins to express, the more successful she will be at maintaining lactation over long periods.[3] Another reason for teaching hand-expression early in the postnatal period is to ensure the mother knows what to do before any problems arise. If a situation then occurs that requires expression, she is already familiar with the principles of expressing by hand, and does not have to learn how to do it at a time when she may be tense, uncomfortable or in pain. Therefore, where the mother may be discharged from hospital care within 24 hours of delivering her baby, she is best taught in this very early period.

3.1.2 How to hand-express

There are several different ways to hand-express. A mother needs to practise and perfect her own technique, although first of all she has to learn the principles underlying the practice, which are basically the same for all mothers. The techniques are refinements, which vary according to individual preference, and which work for some mothers and not for others.

It is important that the mother achieves success at hand-expression from the beginning, because it teaches her many more skills than simply removing milk from the breast. For example, if hand-expression is taught before the baby is able to feed from the breast, then the mother is able to hold and support her breast in an appropriate way to help the baby become attached when he is ready.

Before a mother hand-expresses she should:

◆ wash her hands and fingernails thoroughly with soap and water (there is no need for her to wash her breasts more than once a day)
◆ have a prepared sterile container for her milk (it is preferable to use a bottle or cup which can then be stored without having to transfer the milk into another container; some mothers may find a wide-necked container useful while still perfecting their expression technique).

The following suggestions may help a mother to be well prepared and successful at the time of expression:

◆ Have a clean damp cloth and paper tissues nearby, for her hands, accidental splashes of milk or spillage.
◆ Have a warm drink prepared.
◆ If parted from her baby, she should have a photograph of him nearby, or a piece of his clothing.
◆ Be as relaxed as possible, listen to music or something that makes her laugh, and sit in a really comfortable chair; have low lighting or a candle burning when expressing in the evening.

◆ Express in a warm room.
◆ Express while in a warm bath.

The principles of hand-expression

1. Place the fingers of one hand under the breast. The little finger can be placed against the chest wall, and the other fingers spread evenly under the breast towards the nipple, supporting the breast.

2. Place the thumb on top of the breast and the first finger on the underside of the breast, so that they are opposite one another. Place the thumb and fingers as far back on the breast as is comfortable, towards the chest wall.

3. Gently 'walk' the thumb and fingers down the breast towards the areola and nipple, feeling the nature of the underlying tissue. As the thumb and first finger approach the areola and nipple the underlying tissue will begin to feel different, perhaps more lumpy or more fibrous in

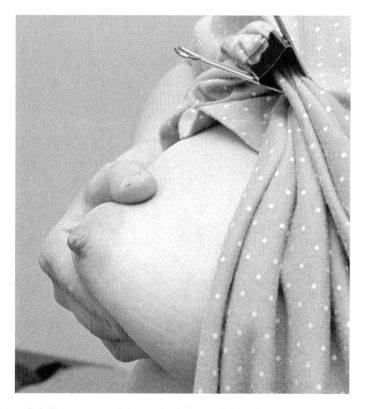

Figure 3.1 The position of the mother's fingers for hand-expression.

nature. This is where the lactiferous sinuses are situated. The margin of the areola is not a good visual guide as to where the sinuses are – but if they cannot be found by feel alone, they are usually situated near the margins of the areola, sometimes within the darkened area and sometimes outside (Fig. 3.1).

4. At the place where the difference is *first* felt, compress and release the breast tissue between the thumb and first finger. Avoid puckering the skin during compression. The action of compression and release should be repeated regularly. The speed, pressure and rhythm of this will vary with each mother, so it is important for her to practise. This action should remove the milk stored in the lactiferous sinuses (Fig. 3.2).

5. To express sufficient milk for a feed, the thumb and forefinger need to move around the outside edge of the lactiferous sinuses to ensure they are all drained.

6. Avoid any sliding movement on the skin; the breasts are extremely sensitive and the skin or underlying tissue can easily be damaged by rough handling.

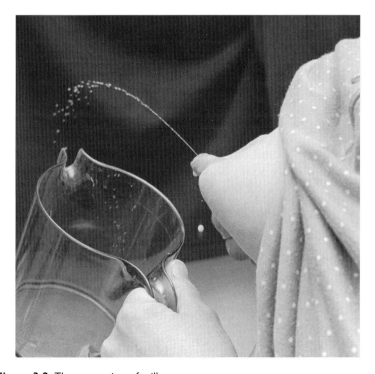

Figure 3.2 The expression of milk.

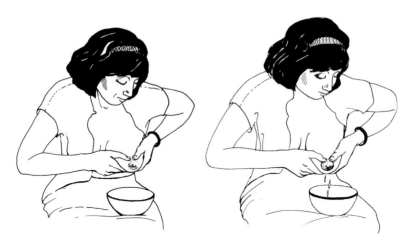

Figure 3.3 Expression of the breast using a two-handed technique.

Advise the mother to always begin hand-expression by 'walking' the thumb and forefinger down the breast, from behind the areola and nipple until she feels the lactiferous sinuses. If she brings her thumb and forefinger from the front, directly onto the nipple and areola, she is more likely to pucker the skin, which makes it difficult to express milk.

Techniques to enhance the success of hand-expression

- ◆ Gently press inwards towards the chest wall when using the compress–release movement. This is easier on a small breast than on a large or pendulous breast.
- ◆ Gentle shaking of the breasts,[4] followed by compression, may help to enhance the milk flow.
- ◆ Use both hands on either side of the breast, rather than only one hand as described above (Fig. 3.3).
- ◆ Place one hand flat on the top of the breast and the other hand flat underneath the breast; without moving the hands, apply simultaneous compress and release movements.
- ◆ Gently roll the thumb or forefinger from side to side towards the nipple. At the same time compress and release, compress and release.

The expression of milk from both breasts at the same time

Milk can be expressed from both breasts at the same time. It can be expressed into a wide-necked container (or two separate containers, one

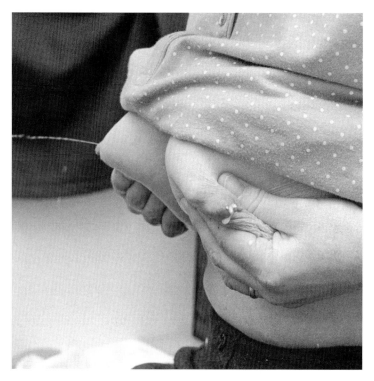

Figure 3.4 Hand-expression from both breasts at the same time (direct the milk flow into a container).

under each breast). The mother should lean forward, with her breasts hanging loosely over the container (Fig. 3.4). This will help in expressing milk from the lobes on the underside of her breasts. The container can be secured between her knees.

There are three main ways of expressing from both breasts at the same time.

1. The breasts can be expressed simultaneously, that is, both breasts being compressed and released at the same time, with frequent pauses to let the lactiferous sinuses in both breasts refill with milk at the same time.

2. The breasts can be expressed alternately, that is, one breast being compressed and released and then the other being compressed and released, switching from side to side. When the milk flow slows or only drips, pause and rest both breasts at the same time for a short period before starting again.

3. The breasts can be expressed alternately, that is one breast is expressed continuously until the milk just drips out and then that breast can pause, meanwhile the other breast is expressed until the milk just drips, then return to the first side. Change sides five or six times until the milk just drips at the start of the expression.

What to expect at an individual expression session

1. With the first few compress–release movements of an expression it is possible that no milk will be immediately visible (particularly in the initial period after birth when colostrum is present).

2. As the movements continue, small amounts of milk will begin to appear at different places on the tip of the nipple.

3. With further compress–release movements, the milk is likely to spurt from the nipple from several different ducts.

4. Gradually the spurts will become less forceful, until there are only drips of milk. The thumb and forefinger should then be moved around the breast to drain the other sinuses.

5. Once the milk flow has slowed to drips, change to the other breast and repeat the above procedure. Continue to alternate between each breast when the milk flow slows. Alternate between each breast five or six times or more.

Initially it may take approximately 1–4 minutes to drain milk from the lactiferous sinuses of each breast, though the time will vary with each mother. Towards the end of the expression the time it takes to remove milk from the lactiferous sinuses is much shorter.

◆ Milk volume will be increased by alternating the expression between the breasts, in the way described in point 5.
◆ Gentle simultaneous hand massage at the time of expression may help with milk flow.

In the first few days of expression, when colostrum is present, it may just drip into a container and not spurt; this is because it is thicker than mature milk. In some mothers the milk never spurts; instead, the milk flow is a steady and consistent stream. This is quite acceptable, although it is important to check that the mother's technique is appropriate for efficient expression.

Some mothers will have colostrum and milk dripping from the nipple before expression begins. This is completely normal and these mothers should be given the information from point 3 of the above sequence of events.

Colostrum is best collected directly from the nipple as it is expressed, using a 1 mL, 2 mL or 5 mL syringe. This ensures that none is lost.

3.1.3 How to teach a mother to hand-express

There are a number of ways to teach a mother the skill of hand-expression:

1. She can be verbally instructed in the principles, by going carefully through each stage.
2. She can be given written instructions.
3. She can be shown what to do using a model breast, by the person teaching, illustrating the movements on her own breast, and getting the mother to copy her, or by using the mother's own breast. All of these ways of teaching the mother work. However, in each case it is helpful to ask the mother to demonstrate on her own breast what she is being taught. If at any point the mother does not understand, ask her if you can show her using her own breast. Sometimes a mother just needs to be shown exactly how to position her fingers, or she may need help to find the lactiferous sinuses. Showing the mother on her own body ensures that she sees how simple the skill of hand-expression is, and knows how it feels for herself. The mother only needs to be touched on this one occasion. Once she has mastered hand-expression and how to position her fingers, the mother is also able, with minimal instruction, to attach her baby to the breast herself, without the need for the baby to be attached to her by someone else. Some mothers may really dislike their breasts being touched, so be very sensitive to their feelings. In this case use a model breast to show the mother exactly the point you are trying to illustrate.

A combination of all three methods is likely to be the most successful. However, whichever way is chosen, it is still important to observe the mother expressing, to be sure she has a safe technique. If the mother does not want to try or be observed, find out how she is getting on within at least 24 hours of being shown. It is useful for the mother to have written instructions for reference.

Practical instruction

If you and the mother decide that the demonstration will be carried out on the mother's own breast, show her what to do initially with your hand on her breast in the exact position she will need to hold her hand. This means standing either slightly behind the mother or to her side (Fig. 3.5). Once you have expressed milk onto her nipple, ask the mother to cover your hand with hers, and then withdraw your hand. The mother's hand should now be in exactly the same position on her breast as your hand was. She can then continue to express from this breast, before initiating the milk flow from the other breast. Once this process has been completed, the mother can be told of the various techniques or

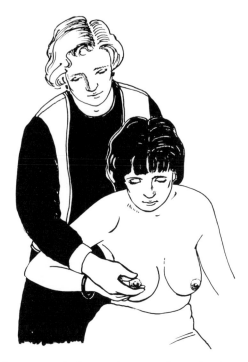

Figure 3.5 Where to stand when teaching a mother to hand-express.

refinements she can add to the basic principles, which she can then practise in her own time.

Practice will perfect the mother's technique of hand-expression. It may not work perfectly the first time she does it. However, it is worth investing time in teaching the principles to the mother and in her acquiring the skill. She will certainly benefit from the help she is given. In circumstances where the mother cannot or does not want to express her milk with a mechanical pump, and she has difficulties with hand-expression, her partner can be taught the skill of hand-expression and help the mother to express her milk.

3.2 EXPRESSION USING A MECHANICAL PUMP

Expression of breastmilk may be necessary in a number of situations, some of which require the mother to express for several weeks; for example, if she has a baby born at less than 27 weeks' gestation. For many mothers, a mechanical pump helps to express breastmilk in sufficient volumes over the many weeks until their babies are able to suckle effectively from the breast. Hand-expression gives the mother a degree of social freedom because it can be done anywhere, with the minimum of equipment or disruption. However, for some mothers, a mechanical means of milk expression is preferable for most everyday use. The following information applies to any mother who needs to use a mechanical pump.

3.2.1 Types of pump

There is a range of pumps available to mothers for hospital use or for use at home. In hospitals the most common pumps are electrically operated. These pumps either use a single funnel connection to remove the milk from one breast at a time, or have two funnel connections so that the milk can be removed simultaneously from both breasts (dual or double pumping). Hand-held pumps, which use batteries or are operated by hand movements, are of many different designs, although they all have a funnel connection at the breast. There is no one type of hand pump that is ideal for all mothers. It is, therefore, particularly valuable if, while the mother is still in hospital and before she is tempted to buy a hand pump, she is given the opportunity to try out a variety of designs which should be available on a unit, to see which pump is most suitable for her needs (they are expensive, especially if once purchased they do not work for her).

Hand pumps and hand-expression are useful if a mother returns to work, or to give her more social freedom.

Which kind of pump to use?

Electric pumps

◆ Electric pumps are easy to use. Once the electricity is switched on and various settings are made the mother is required only to hold the bottle and funnel to her breast (Fig. 3.6).

◆ Many mothers are able to express more milk than their babies require, particularly in the first few days and weeks. Gradually mothers may notice a reduction in the amount of milk they express; at this point they should increase the number of times they express. The mother's aim should be to meet her baby's daily milk requirements.

◆ Dual or double pumping may reduce the time spent in expressing, and for some mothers the volume of milk produced is higher than with single pumping. Some mothers, however, find this method uncomfortable and awkward to do.

◆ To use the pump the mother must have access to an electricity supply, so if this is her only method of expression she may have to

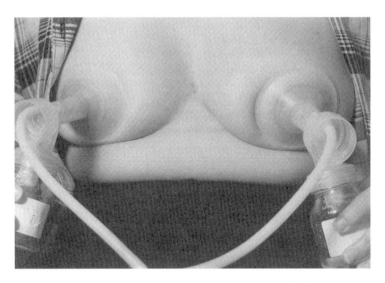

Figure 3.6 Expression using a pump with an attachment for double-pumping (photograph courtesy of the North Staffs Neonatal Unit).

arrange her days, and where she is, around the times she needs to express.

◆ Some of the newer electric pumps are fairly small and lightweight, but even so they are not easily portable. A mother who may be away from the hospital or from her home for longer than 2–3 hours may find hand-expression, or a battery- or hand-operated pump, useful as well. There is no reason not to use different methods according to need.

◆ Some mothers may find their milk does not flow easily with an electric pump.

Battery-operated pumps

◆ Battery-operated pumps are also easy to use.
◆ The battery is often situated in such a position that mothers may not have a clear view of the milk flowing into the bottle. A mirror may be helpful in this case if the mother finds this type of pump the right one for her.

Hand-operated pumps

◆ There are several types of hand-operated pumps. In hospitals the 'syringe' design is commonly available. This design of pump can be used when the breasts are full, but is difficult to use when the breasts are soft.

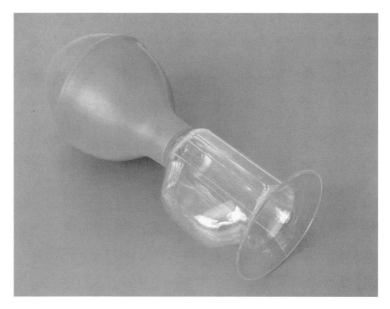

Figure 3.7 A 'bicycle horn' pump.

◆ Some hand pumps have a lever or compression mechanism requiring repetitive hand movements to make them work.
◆ All hand-operated pumps can be tiring for the mother to use, which can affect the efficiency of milk removal.

'Bicycle horn' style pumps (Fig. 3.7) should *not* be used for milk expression. They are difficult to keep clean or sterilize because of the rubber bulb part of the pump. These pumps may be useful for expressing a little milk from an engorged breast, when hand-expression is not possible because the breast is too firm. Only partially squeeze the bulb so that the suction is not too fierce. The milk expressed should be discarded.

Because there is no similarity between using a mechanical breast-pump and breastfeeding, a mother may need to adopt some of the following strategies to help maintain her milk supply over long periods of time. A mother who is expressing her milk by hand may also find this information of use.

3.2.2 How to pump

Once the basic method of using an electric or hand pump is explained to a mother, there are several tips that may help her maintain her supply and make expression more comfortable.

◆ Expression in a warm room will be beneficial. The mother may find placing a warm cloth over the breast may also help with milk flow.

◆ Expressing from one breast while the baby is feeding from the other may help a mother who has a diminished milk supply.

◆ Hand-expression of breastmilk is a more physiological technique than mechanical expression, and there is evidence to suggest that it results in higher prolactin levels than ordinary single mechanical expression,[5,6] although less than with dual pumping. A combination of methods may be a useful compromise, with mechanical pumping performed for the first 5–10 minutes, and then expression by hand until there is no further milk flow. Any combination can be used, as long as it is satisfactory to the mother.

◆ Breast massage will help encourage milk flow if performed prior to expression.

◆ Alternating the pumping of each breast every 2–4 minutes is shown to encourage and increase the flow.

◆ Using a flexi-shield (Fig. 3.8). For some mothers this device provides a more comfortable means of expression than using the glass or plastic funnel on its own. The shield fits on to the rim of the funnel, and

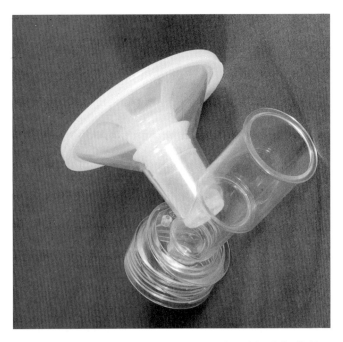

Figure 3.8 The flexi-shield (photograph courtesy of the North Staffs Neonatal Unit and Egnell-Ameda).

allows the mother to use the highest setting on the breastpump, which provides a more effective rhythm of expression.

◆ The position of the funnel at the breast, when expressing, should be slightly changed at regular intervals to stimulate different lobes.

◆ Dual or double pumping with an electric pump allows expression to be completed more quickly (see Fig. 3.6). It may be beneficial to have 30-second to 60-second pauses during the session every 3–4 minutes, so that milk can drain into the lactiferous sinuses (this occurs where a pump does not have a pause mechanism built into it). Dual or double pumping is reported to encourage an increased milk supply and high prolactin levels when compared with other methods of expression.[7] Mothers who hand-express may also express from both breasts at the same time.

Whichever method of breast expression the mother finds most comfortable, successful and acceptable should be used.

3.3 GENERAL INFORMATION FOR HAND OR PUMP EXPRESSION OF BREASTMILK

As with hand-expression, it is important for the mother who uses a pump to begin expressing her milk as early as possible, preferably within the first 6 hours of delivery and certainly within the first 24 hours. This usually results in improved quantities of milk being expressed in comparison with mothers who begin expression only on the third or fourth day.[3] This also applies to a mother who has had a caesarean section, unless there are good medical contraindications to early expression. Following caesarean delivery it may be necessary for the midwife or neonatal nurse to initiate and carry out the first few expressions until the mother is feeling well enough to express her own breastmilk. It is important to check which drugs the mother has been given and whether they may adversely affect the breastmilk. Even if they do, the expression should still be commenced early to stimulate milk production – but the milk may need to be discarded at first.

The colostrum obtained in the first few days should be given to the baby immediately, or at the earliest opportunity after expression, preferably as a bolus feed, for it has many medicinal qualities.[8–10] Colostrum is best collected directly as it is expressed from the breast. Hand-expression is the best method because of the small quantities of colostrum produced; it can be collected in a small syringe.

3.3.1 How often?

To ensure an adequate milk supply over any length of time, expression should be maintained every 2–3 hours for a minimum of six to eight times in 24 hours.[3] Often more frequent expression is necessary – ten to twelve times in 24 hours, particularly if the milk supply begins to diminish.

Expression should be started soon after the mother gets up in the morning and, to ensure the gap is not too long overnight, it should be one of the last things she does before going to bed. The other expressions should be spaced equally throughout the day. Ideally the mother should express at least once during the night as well.[5] While she is in hospital it is the mother, and not the staff, who should make the decision whether she is to be woken to express milk or to feed her baby. However, she needs to understand why it is important for her to express at night, and not to go for longer than 6–7 hours without expressing. It is not uncommon for mothers to have uncomfortably full breasts by the morning, particularly in the early postnatal period. If this occurs regularly, the mother's milk production may decline owing to the feedback inhibitor of lactation.

3.3.2 How long?

Length of expression will vary between each mother but will commonly take 10–20 minutes for each breast. On the first day a few minutes only on each side may be as much as the mother can tolerate. A time limit should not be specified, however, and she should be advised to express her milk until the flow ceases. The expression of both breasts should not normally take longer than an hour. If this is happening, the way the mother is expressing her milk needs to be checked. If the mother is using an electric pump, she should start with the pump on the lowest settings and gradually increase the suction.

3.3.3 The amount of milk produced

The amount of milk produced at each expression will vary throughout the day. The greatest volume is usually obtained in the morning, with lower volumes expressed as the day proceeds. The volume may also vary according to the emotional state of the mother. In a neonatal or paediatric unit, for example, the baby's clinical condition may be unstable, causing the mother to be very stressed at times. Few mothers are aware of the normal differences in the diurnal milk flow and fewer still are aware that any emotional upset may temporarily reduce their milk flow (an effect frequently observed on neonatal units). It is important that the mother is aware of this, so that she does not worry unnecessarily about her ability to lactate.

Colostrum appears to be produced in very small volumes, often no more than 1–10 mL per expression. For the needs of most term babies this is quite sufficient in the first few days after delivery and additional fluids are not normally required. This will apply, for example, if a baby is receiving prophylactic antibiotics but is otherwise well – as in the case of a term baby whose mother suffered premature rupture of the membranes. This baby will not require additional fluids.

A mother expressing her own breastmilk may notice:

◆ The milk flow increases substantially over the first few days after birth, with the daily variation in milk volume obtained at each expression becoming more obvious (see section 1.4 of Chapter 1).

◆ The milk supply may begin to diminish at around 10–14 days, particularly if the mother has been staying in hospital with her baby from birth. This period often coincides with a change in the mother's routine; for example, she may go home from hospital, her partner may go back to work, she may become more active. This reduction may be more noticeable in a mother using an electric pump.

Some mothers who use both hand-expression and an electric pump to collect their milk may notice that they obtain greater quantities of milk with the pump than by hand. This is quite common. Milk that is expressed by hand until no more milk can be obtained will have the right balance of nutrients for the baby. It is important, however, that the mother does not time the length of expression or she may not have enough of the fat-rich hind-milk in her expressed milk. Some mothers who cannot express sufficient quantities of milk for their babies by electric pump may conversely find that they can produce increased amounts by hand. If this is the case they should be encouraged to continue with hand-expression for as long as possible. Some mothers may find hand-expression takes longer than expression by electric pump.

As long as the mother continues to receive **constant support and reassurance**, she should be able to maintain her milk supply for as long as she wants to, regardless of whether she is expressing by hand or pump. **Most mothers are quite capable of expressing the amount of milk their babies require**. It is really worth emphasizing to the mother that she should seek support and accept **all** offers of help if she is at home, especially if she has other children to care for. It will be hard for her to find enough hours in the day to express, visit her baby, and maintain family and household tasks. Consistent support is crucial.

3.4 HOW TO STOP USING A PUMP

A mother who is about to stop expressing her milk by mechanical pump should wean off the pump gradually rather than suddenly stop. This is particularly important where she has consistently produced more milk than her baby needs. Gradual weaning from the pump gives the breasts time to respond naturally to her baby's requirements. This process appears to take a few days, if the mother has been using a pump for several weeks.

When a mother suddenly stops using a mechanical pump the milk may not be removed in sufficient quantities by her baby. This can lead to engorgement and, if it occurs continually, to a diminished milk supply and to mastitis.

3.4.1 Weaning off the pump

Weaning off the pump is particularly important for any mother who has been expressing by mechanical pump for 2 weeks or more, or who expresses more milk than her baby needs.

1. Weaning off the pump should take place over a period of 4–5 days, not abruptly.
2. If possible the process should be completed while the baby is still in a hospital unit. It therefore needs to be commenced approximately 5–6 days prior to the baby's discharge.
3. The milk expressed can be given by cup if required, or stored.
4. The amount of milk to be expressed depends upon the mother's milk supply.
5. Write down the regimen to be used by the mother.
6. Expression should be completed before breastfeeding takes place, so that the baby receives the fat-rich hind-milk.
7. Expression by hand will help the mother reduce her milk production.

3.4.2 A sample regimen

The volumes used in this sample regimen are intended as examples only. How much breastmilk an individual mother expresses prior to each breastfeeding session will depend upon how much milk she was expressing before the establishment of breastfeeding began.

Day 1

◆ Express 20–30 mL of breastmilk in total from both breasts, i.e. 10–15 mL from each breast, in the morning before breastfeeding.
◆ Express 15–25 mL of breastmilk in total, in the afternoon before breastfeeding.
◆ Express 10–20 mL of breastmilk in total, in the evening before breastfeeding.

It is important to use hand-expression or a hand pump to express these amounts. Do not use an electric pump as this will usually maintain or increase production, not reduce it.

Day 2–5

Express as for day 1, but each day *reduce* the amounts expressed by:

◆ 5 mL of breastmilk in the morning
◆ 2–3 mL of breastmilk in the afternoon and evening.

Day 6

Do not express any milk before feeding from the breast.

After completing this weaning process the mother should be producing quantities of milk closer to those her baby needs. However, this regimen can be repeated if the baby does not continue to gain weight steadily, or if his weight becomes static or falls slightly. To repeat the regimen, reduce the amount of breastmilk expressed in the sample regimen by approximately 5 mL at each expression, as follows.

Day 1

◆ Express 15–20 mL of breastmilk in the morning rather than 20–30 mL.
◆ Express 10–20 mL of breastmilk in the afternoon.
◆ Express 5–15 mL of breastmilk in the evening.

Days 2–5

Reduce the expressions of day 2–5 by 5 mL at each expression.

3.5 STORAGE OF EXPRESSED BREASTMILK AND ITS SEQUENCE OF USE

3.5.1 Containers and storage

Containers for expressed breastmilk to be given to babies on neonatal or paediatric units

1. A sterile container **specially designed** for expressed breastmilk should always be used for milk collection and storage.[11]

2. Glass or plastic (polypropylene or polycarbonate) bottles are **recommended**. Plastic bags, including those designated for breastmilk collection, stainless steel or plastic containers found at home, such as yoghurt pots, **should not be used**.

3. Small 1 mL, 2 mL or 5 mL sterile syringes are ideal for collecting colostrum. These can be spigoted to protect the colostrum from contamination.

4. In hospital a mother should have a new collecting set (i.e. bottle, funnel and tubing) for each expression to reduce the possibility of cross-infection.[7]

5. At home the mother should, whenever possible, use sterile containers provided by the hospital. If she has to sterilize containers herself, she should follow the instructions given on sterilization procedures by the hospital (if a chemical disinfectant is to be used). A domestic steam sterilizer can be used by the mother.

6. Before a container or any expression equipment is sterilized or disinfected, the mother should wash it with detergent and hot water, using a bottle-brush, followed by thorough rinsing.

Fewer bacteria are found in hand-expressed milk than in mechanically expressed milk,[12] which reflects possible contamination from the equipment. This emphasizes the importance of ensuring that any breastpump equipment used is properly cleaned and sterilized.

Expression and storage

1. When a mother expresses her milk into a bottle it should not be filled right to the top. At least 2.5 cm should be left so that if the milk is frozen, it can expand without the bottle breaking.

2. Whenever possible, milk should be stored in quantities roughly equivalent to the amount the baby requires for each feed. This may mean the amount expressed needs to be divided into more than one container if the amount expressed is far more than the baby requires. If the amount is less than 90 mL, stir the contents first before dividing it into separate containers. This ensures equal distribution of the fore-milk and hind-milk. If more than 100 mL is expressed and the baby requires much less, follow the instructions in Chapter 5, section 5.3.2.

3. Each bottle should be clearly labelled with the mother's name, and date and time of expression.

4. Freshly expressed breastmilk can be left at room temperature for 6 hours,[13,14] although if it is not to be used immediately it should be refrigerated as soon as possible.

5. Raw breastmilk (i.e. milk that has not been pasteurized) that will be used within 48 hours should be stored in the refrigerator at 2–4 °C.[11,15]

6. Breastmilk that is not to be used within 24 hours should be stored in the freezer at −20 °C. It can be stored for a maximum of 3 months, if it is to be fed to a preterm baby. After this time it should be discarded.

7. There is little evidence either for or against giving milk that is more than 3 months old to well, older babies.

The effect of the container on milk composition

Containers used to store breastmilk should ideally be made of glass or plastic. Although not recommended for storage, stainless steel containers, plastic bags designed for breastmilk, and various other plastic containers are often used. Several studies have reported that the type of container can affect the milk composition. Constituents of the milk may stick to the sides of the containers: for example, lipids (fats)[16] and secretory immunoglobulin A (sIgA)[17] have been observed to stick to plastic storage bags. These bags also have a tendency to leak, increasing the likelihood of bacterial contamination. There is an acknowledged loss of immunoglobulins from milk stored in stainless steel containers.[11] Plastic containers not designed for breastmilk storage may be difficult to sterilize adequately.

Concern has also been expressed about plastic bottles. The repeated cleaning of containers made of polypropylene can increase the risk of bacterial contamination from scratches to the inside of the container.[17]

Glass containers are recommended for storing expressed breastmilk. They do not appear to have any adverse effect on the milk constituents and, although cells have been observed to stick to the sides of glass, they have also been observed to detach from the sides after 24 hours of storage.[17] Glass containers can be easily cleaned, thus reducing the risk of contamination.

3.5.2 Defrosting breastmilk

1. Defrosting raw breastmilk is best achieved by putting the bottle of frozen milk into the refrigerator.[11] It can also be thawed at room temperature, though once thawed it should be either used or put in a refrigerator.

2. Defrosted milk should be discarded after 12 hours in a refrigerator.[11]

3. Frozen milk can also be defrosted by putting the bottle in running warm water.[18] The cap should not be loosened until the milk has thawed and the bottle has been dried.

4. When removed from the freezer, the container should be labelled with the date and time. The milk should be used within 12 hours. Freezing destroys many of the cells in breastmilk and therefore affects its anti-infective properties, making it more susceptible to bacterial growth if kept for longer periods.

5. Defrosting breastmilk in a microwave is not recommended, as this may heat the milk unevenly with a potential risk of burning the baby's mouth and throat. Microwaving also destroys 30% of the protective immunoproteins.[18]

Do not refreeze milk once it is defrosted!

3.5.3 Sequence of breastmilk use

1. Use all colostrum.
2. Use the first 14 days of milk in order (there is still colostrum in this milk).
3. After this, use milk as it is produced, i.e. use fresh milk if possible or use the milk produced on the same day.
4. Where a mother produces more milk than her baby requires, use the milk in order of expression for that day, and freeze the remainder, i.e. use the milk she produces in the morning before the milk produced in the afternoon or evening. The highest fat levels are generally found in breastmilk expressed in the morning and early afternoon,[19] therefore this milk should be given to the baby.

3.6 PROLONGED EXPRESSION OF BREASTMILK

Any mother who has to express her milk for longer than 3 days will need some of the following information in addition to that given above. The information at the end of this section is particularly important for any mother who has to express her breastmilk over a period of weeks, rather than days.

Prolonged expression of milk may be necessary if a mother wishes to provide her own breastmilk for a preterm, ill or bottle-fed baby. A number of potential problems can occur, depending upon the length of time over which the mother has to maintain her lactation. Her success depends upon a level of commitment that is sometimes difficult to sustain, together with the support of her family, hospital staff and anyone else involved in her care.

3.6.1 Suggestions for reducing long-term problems

The following suggestions are aimed at reducing long-term problems that may arise from the prolonged expression of breastmilk.

◆ Advise the mother to express milk when she is in the unit with her baby, or in an atmosphere in which she can relax, listening to music, or with a photograph of her baby beside her.

◆ Whenever possible, it is worth reminding the mother that, as each day passes, her baby is either becoming more mature, growing and getting stronger, or (if he is recovering from an illness) getting better. This brings breastfeeding closer and the prospect of the baby being able to stimulate his mother's milk supply on his own.

◆ It is worth a mother experimenting with different methods of expressing to find the one most appropriate for her. It may be that the

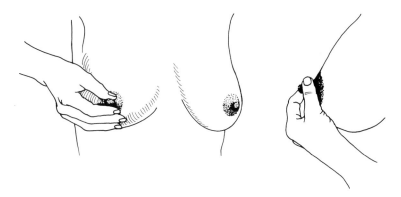

Figure 3.9 Nipple stimulation using the thumb and forefinger.

method she is using is not the best for her and this may be causing – or appearing to cause – a diminished milk supply.

◆ Massage of the breasts prior to expression for 3–5 minutes will stimulate the blood supply and may therefore encourage the milk supply.

◆ Very gentle massage of the nipple for half a minute may stimulate the release of prolactin and oxytocin, and therefore help with the milk production and let-down reflex. The nipple can either be rolled gently between the thumb and forefinger (Fig. 3.9), or the palm of the hand can be gently moved back and forth over the tip of the nipple. If the mother's partner can stimulate the nipple the result may be much faster!

◆ Encourage the mother's partner or a friend to massage her back. It is suggested that this may help stimulate the release of oxytocin and the let-down reflex.[20]

◆ Hand-expression is a useful and tactile method of expressing and should be used whenever possible. If the mother uses an electric pump, encourage her to hand-express after she thinks that she has finished on the pump. She will almost certainly see that she still has milk and, if she can become proficient in expressing this, it is nutritionally very important for her baby.

◆ Suggest to the mother that she keeps a record of the amounts that she expresses. She may well be encouraged to see that she has more milk than she thinks she has. If her milk supply has diminished, she may see a positive result from the advice given to her.

◆ If or when the mother's milk does begin to diminish, reassure her that this is not a permanent state and urge her to continue expressing. Increasing the number of sessions of expression may help to increase her milk supply.

◆ While it cannot be emphasized enough how important regular expressing is, it is necessary to accept that the mother needs to have an occasional break. She can safely miss an expression provided she does so only rarely. Indeed, it is important she does take a break. If she is to be able to go out and still maintain regular expression, she may find the electric pump useful at home, and hand-expression useful when she is out.

3.7 BACK MASSAGE

There are several methods of back massage. The following three methods are easy to do and can involve a partner. They are also reported to be pleasant for the mother. It may be advisable for a mother to have a container nearby or placed on her lap as milk will sometimes begin to flow spontaneously during back massage. Always finish a massage by gently placing the hands palm down on either side of the upper back for a few seconds; this signals to the mother that the massage has ended.

3.7.1 Method I

Although it is possible to do this massage over clothing, friction can make the skin on the knuckles very raw. It is better to use a little body oil directly on the skin of the back. If aromatherapy or homoeopathic products are preferred, it is advisable to consult a qualified practitioner.

1. The mother should sit down, fold her arms in front of her on a table, and rest her head on her arms. Her back should be exposed.
2. The massage is performed on either side of the spinal column, from the base of the neck to just below the shoulder blades.
3. The person conducting the massage should form her hands into fists. The knuckles of one fist at the top of the mother's back, and the other fist just below the mother's shoulder blade on the opposite side (Fig. 3.10).
4. The knuckles should either be facing each other or at right angles to the spinal column.
5. Using fairly brisk movements, move the fists in opposite directions, i.e. with one fist beginning at the top of the back and moving firmly to just below the shoulder blades and the other fist beginning at just below the shoulder blades and moving to the top of the back.
6. Continue for about 3–4 minutes, or for however long is acceptable to the mother and the masseur!

3.7.2 Method 2

1. The mother should sit down, fold her arms in front of her on a table, and rest her head on her arms.
2. The person conducting the massage uses her thumbs, one placed on either side of the spinal column at the top of the mother's back (Fig. 3.11).

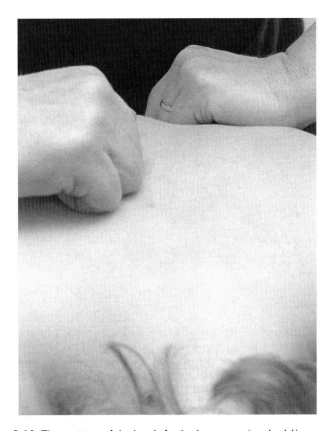

Figure 3.10 The position of the hands for back massage (method 1).

3. Using firm pressure, small, slow circular movements should be made with the thumbs.
4. Both sides of the spine are massaged at the same time, from the base of the neck to just below the shoulder blades.
5. Continue for about 3–4 minutes or for however long is acceptable.

3.7.3 Method 3

This is a very simple massage.

1. The mother should sit leaning forward with her head resting on her crossed arms.
2. Place one hand flat in the middle of the mother's back, level with the base of the neck, covering the spinal column.
3. Place the other hand just below the shoulder blades, flat in the middle of the back covering the spinal column.

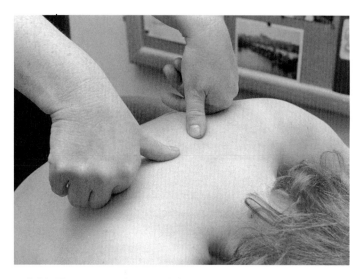

Figure 3.11 The position of the hands for back massage (method 2).

4. Using firm, smooth strokes, slide the hand at the top of the back down to the other hand.
5. Swap hands, and begin again. Continue in this way for several minutes.

3.8 BREAST MASSAGE

Breast massage complements hand-expression. There are several ways to massage, all equally successful. In a neonatal unit, it is important to teach a mother a method that is gentle and will not damage the skin or underlying tissues. This is particularly important when massage may be used long-term.

3.8.1 Why is it helpful?

◆ It helps a mother to relax. If she is feeling tired, anxious or has a poor milk supply, 4–5 minutes of gentle massage before a feed or expression will help to calm her, and focus her mind on her milk.
◆ It is easy for a partner to learn and do.
◆ It is easy to massage while feeding or expressing, to encourage the milk flow.
◆ Oxytocin is released.[21]
◆ There is some evidence to suggest that if gentle nipple stimulation is also used with the massage, it may help improve a diminished

milk supply (by increased prolactin release, particularly if performed prior to mechanical pumping or hand-expression).[22] Sometimes nipple stimulation alone will result in milk beginning to flow from the breast.

◆ It encourages a good blood flow to the breast and may therefore encourage an efficient milk supply.[23]

◆ It enables mothers to recognize early signs of breast engorgement, or blocked ducts or lobes.

◆ It effectively helps disperse engorged lobes and mastitis.

3.8.2 How to massage

There are no right or wrong ways to massage. Some methods may be more successful than others, but it is important to be gentle, particularly if the technique favoured by a mother involves moving her hands over the skin of her breast. The 'whole hand' and the 'fist' method can be performed over clothing using only one hand. This can be useful if the mother has other small children who want to be cuddled or read to at the same time.

Teaching a mother about breast massage provides an ideal opportunity to teach her the principles of **breast self-examination**, as one of the simplest methods of breast massage uses the same hand movements.

The 'whole hand' method

1. The mother places her hand flat on the top of the breast as in Fig. 3.12. Either hand can be used.

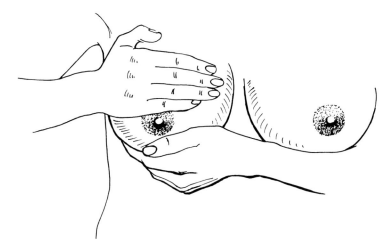

Figure 3.12 The 'whole hand' method of breast massage.

2. She should then raise the outer side of her hand, so that only the thumb and first finger side of her hand are left in contact with the breast.
3. She should then roll her hand back to its original position using a firm movement, her fingers together and moved first.
4. Through her fingers she will feel the nature of the underlying tissue. This should cause no pain.
5. She should move her hand around the breast.
6. To massage the underside of the breast the mother should support the weight of her breast in the palm of her hand. Using her fingers together she should move them in the same way as already described.
7. She should always move her hand towards the areola and nipple.

Mothers with large, heavy breasts may need to use the second hand to support the breast as illustrated in Fig. 3.12. Using this method a mother can detect a blocked duct before it becomes obvious. No damage from friction can occur.

The 'fist' method

This method is useful prior to a feed or expression, because it enables all lobes of the breast to be massaged, and can be performed using only one hand without the need to remove any clothing. Either hand can be used according to ease. In addition no damage from friction can occur. This method originated in Papua New Guinea.

1. Form the hand into a fist, place the thumb end at the top of the breast towards the chest wall. Hold the fist at right angles to the chest (Fig. 3.13a).

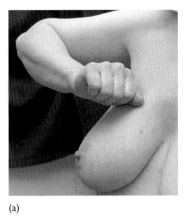
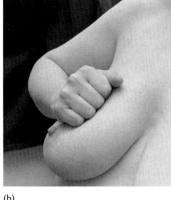

(a)   (b)

Figure 3.13 The 'fist' method of breast massage.

2. Using a rolling action, roll the fist down the breast towards the nipple, transferring the pressure as this is done. Never roll in the opposite direction, because this will interfere with efficient breast drainage (Fig. 3.13b).
3. When massaging lobes under the breast, place the little-finger end of the fist at the chest wall and roll the fist upwards towards the nipple. If the breast is large or pendulous, an alternative way is to use a flat hand. Place the little finger next to the chest wall and gently roll the palm of the hand towards the nipple.
4. The pressure should be firm but gentle. If it is painful, stop and apply less pressure. It should be comfortable. It is very easy and effective.

It is very helpful if the mother is shown how to massage. It is preferable if you can demonstrate the different methods on your own body and then ask the mother to copy you. Tell her to be gentle but firm. It is difficult to massage the mother's breast with your hand.

Other methods of massage

◆ Using the fingertips, lightly tap the breast in a 'dancing' motion. Use a circular movement around the breast, or move the fingers from the edges of the breast to the areola in straight lines, gradually working all around the breast (Fig. 3.14).

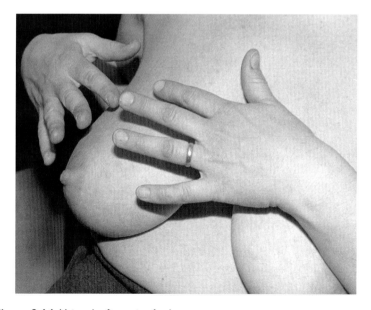

Figure 3.14 Using the fingertips for breast massage.

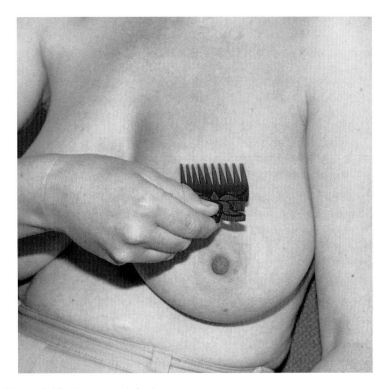

Figure 3.15 Using a comb for breast massage.

◆ Use a wide-toothed comb (Fig. 3.15) or fingertips to stroke the breast gently from the edges of the breast to the areola.
◆ Use a feather!

The 'finger' method for blocked lobes or ducts

The following 'finger' method of massage is specifically to help disperse a blocked lobe or duct. This method is also performed using only one hand and should be used directly on the skin of the breast rather than over clothing.

1. The first two fingers of the hand are used for the opposite breast, so that the right hand massages the left breast (Fig. 3.16).
2. Starting near the chest wall, locate the blocked lobe or duct and then lightly press the first two fingers gently into the breast tissue, making small circular movements over the blocked area, without moving the fingers over the skin.
3. Gradually move the fingers towards the areola along the full length of the blockage.

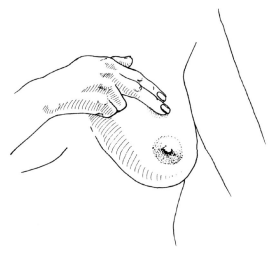

Figure 3.16 The 'finger' method of breast massage, for blocked ducts and mastitis.

4. Gently vibrating the fingers during the massage may make it more effective.
5. If the breast is large, use all four fingers.

This should be followed by hand-expression.

3.9 EXPRESSING FOR ONE-OFF SOCIAL EVENTS

There will always be occasions, once the baby has been discharged from hospital, that the mother may wish or need to go out and return after her baby has fed. It is worth expressing some milk in preparation for these events well in advance, and storing the milk. A mother can begin to express and store some milk whenever she wants to. If the baby is able to breastfeed from the time of birth it is better to wait until after the fourth day, so that the baby receives as much of the colostrum as possible. After that, if a mother feels she has some milk left after a feed, or if her baby only fed from one side and the other side feels full, any milk she can then express can be stored. It is best to store milk in feed-size quantities to minimize the amount of waste after defrosting. Some mothers use ice cube trays with a lid. A mother can express a small amount into a container and freeze it; when she next expresses, as long as she allows the amount to cool, she can add it to the frozen milk. This is best used for a well baby, not a preterm or ill baby.

3.10 SUPPLEMENTARY AND REPLACEMENT FEEDING

A term, healthy baby should require no supplementary feeds (i.e. no extra fluids in addition to feeding from the breast); the baby should be fed on demand. Night feeds are particularly important and a baby should be given to the mother to breastfeed, rather than be given a replacement feed (i.e. a total feed in place of feeding from the breast) so that she can sleep. Only if there is a very good medical reason for not waking her should demand breastfeeding be interrupted.

Term babies admitted to a neonatal unit who are capable of feeding on demand, come into this category. They include:

◆ babies receiving antibiotic therapy or phototherapy
◆ low-birthweight babies (i.e. less than 2500 g at birth), who are awake and hungry, with a satisfactory blood glucose level.

There is no reason for these babies to have replacement feeding or supplementary feeding. Giving supplementary or replacement feeds can lead to the mother's own milk supply decreasing. This also applies where rigid timing between feeds does not allow a baby to feed when ready, particularly if formula milk is used as the supplement. If a baby is hungry the breast should be given, even if this is not at the time scheduled on a feeding chart. In hot weather, there is no evidence that supplementary feeding is necessary. Breastfeeding provides sufficient fluid for a term baby's needs.[24]

3.10.1 When supplementary or replacement feeds are necessary

There are situations in which a baby will need supplementary or replacement feeds. These are listed below. It is preferable to use a mother's own expressed milk, rather than a formula milk.

1. If a baby is preterm and unable to take a full feed from the breast he will require supplementary feeding via a nasogastric or orogastric tube or cup. This usually applies to a baby who is just beginning to learn to breastfeed and only suckles for a short time. As the baby becomes more efficient at the breast, less milk will need to be given by tube or cup and fewer supplementary feeds will be needed.

It is impossible to suggest a regimen which is suitable in all cases because each individual baby is so different. Some preterm or sick babies will breastfeed well on one occasion in the day and require no supplementary feeds, while the same baby on another occasion will feed only for a few minutes and need a supplement. Some babies will not feed again for the rest of the day and require complete replacement feeds. If a well, preterm baby has taken a satisfactory breastfeed, i.e. audible swallow sounds are heard and the mother's breasts are comfortable after the feed, and her baby settles well afterwards, a supplement should not be necessary. Similarly, if the baby wakes and appears hungry after 1½–2 hours, the breast should be offered again before any attempt at supplementation is made.

The mother should be encouraged to express her breastmilk so that she has some milk in the refrigerator or freezer, which can be used for a supplementary or replacement feed. If a baby goes to the breast for part of a feed the mother should express both breasts afterwards. This milk can then be used for the next feed if required.

2. A very sleepy, jaundiced baby may need supplementation via a nasogastric or orogastric tube, or a cup, if regular breastfeeds are not possible. This is usually only necessary for a short time. The mother should express during this period, but the baby should always be offered the breast before supplementation. Unless the jaundiced baby is also preterm, replacement feeds are unlikely to be required.

3. Supplementation or replacement feeding of an ill baby, whether term or preterm, may be required until the baby is strong or well enough to sustain his nutritive needs totally from the breast. The baby should be held next to the breast whenever possible so that if he does want to breastfeed, he has the opportunity; a gastric tube feed can be given at the same time. The mother should be reassured that once an ill baby is better, feeding from the breast will improve. Similarly, if the baby is preterm, as he matures his feeding will also improve. The mother may need to be very patient.

In any situation where a supplement is considered necessary but there is insufficient expressed breastmilk, always try to mix some mother's milk with the formula milk – this enhances the digestion of the formula milk.

Always make sure supplementary feeds are really necessary!

3.11 BREAST SHELLS AND DRIP CATCHERS

Drip catchers should only be used to collect drip milk at the time of feeding. If worn between feeds, they can create pressure on the lactiferous sinuses, and cause subsequent blockage and mastitis. Mothers rarely wear brassières that have sufficient extra room for either a shell or drip catcher.

There is no evidence to show that breast shells (Fig. 3.17) improve the protractility of a flat or inverted nipple in the antenatal period.[25]

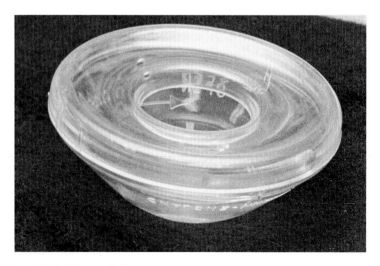

Figure 3.17 A breast shell.

3.12 MILK BANKS

A mother who has more breastmilk than her baby requires can donate the excess to a milk bank. The milk is heat-treated and stored until it is needed.

In the UK there are 14 milk banks. They vary in size; some serve large areas, while others serve a particular hospital. Many more are needed to ensure that all babies in neonatal and paediatric units can benefit from receiving human milk if their mothers are unable or choose not to breastfeed.

More information about milk banking can be obtained from the United Kingdom Association for Milk Banking (see the Appendix).

REFERENCES

1. Lang S, Lawrence CJ, L'E Orme R (1994) Sodium in hand and pump expressed human breastmilk. *Early Hum Dev* **38**: 131–138.
2. World Health Organization (1989) Infant feeding: the physiological basis. *WHO Bull* **67** (suppl.): 76–77.
3. Hopkinson JM, Schanler RJ, Garza C (1988) Milk production by mothers of preterm infants. *Pediatrics* **81**: 815–819.
4. Marmet C (1985) *Manual Expression of Breast Milk – Marmet Technique.* Reprint no. 27. Franklin Park: La Leche League International.
5. Zinaman MJ, Hughes V, Queenan JT et al (1992) Acute prolactin and oxytocin responses and milk yields to infant suckling and artificial methods of expression in lactating women. *Pediatrics* **89**: 437–440.

6. Howie PJ, McNeilly AS, McArdle T et al (1980) The relationship between suckling-induced prolactin response and lactogenesis. *J Clin Endocrinol Metabol* **50**: 670–673.
7. Auerbach KG (1990) Sequential and simultaneous breastpumping: a comparison. *Int J Nutr Stud* **27**: 257–265.
8. Mathur NB, Dwarkadas AM, Sharma VK et al (1990) Anti-infective factors in preterm human colostrum. *Acta Paediatr Scand* **79**: 1039–1044.
9. Jannson L, Karlson FA, Westermark B (1985) Mitogenic activity and epidermal growth factor content in human milk. *Acta Paediatr Scand* **74**: 250–253.
10. Cure in a mother's milk. *New Scientist* 20 April 1991.
11. United Kingdom Association for Milk Banking (2001) *Guidelines for the collection, storage and handling of breast milk for a mother's own baby on a neonatal unit,* 2nd ed. London: UKAMB.
12. Sosa R, Barness L (1987) Bacterial growth in refrigerated human milk. *Am J Dis Child* **141**: 111–112.
13. Pittard WB, Anderson DM, Cerutti ERC et al (1985) Bacteriological qualities of human milk. *J Pediatr* **107**: 240–243.
14. Nwankwo MU, Offor R, Okolo AA et al (1988) Bacterial growth in expressed breast milk. *Ann Trop Paediatr* **8**: 92–95.
15. Jensen R, Jenson G (1992) Speciality lipids for infant nutrition. 1. Milks and formulas. *J Pediatr Gastroenterol Nutr* **15**: 232–245.
16. Ellis L, Hamosh M (1991) Human milk: stability of digestive enzymes in expressed milk. In: *Human Lactation V: Mechanisms Regulating Lactation and Infant Nutrient Utilisation.* Picciano MF, Lonnerdal B (eds). Chichester: John Wiley, pp. 389–393.
17. Hopkinson J, Garza C, Asquith MT (1990) Human milk storage in glass containers. *J Hum Lact* **6**: 104–105.
18. Sigman M, Burke KL, Swarner OW (1989) Effects of microwaving human milk: changes in IgA content and bacterial count. *J Am Diet Assoc* **89**: 690–692.
19. Lammi-Keefe CJ, Ferris AM, Jensen RG (1990) Changes in human milk at 0600, 1000, 1400, 1800, and 2200 h. *J Pediatr Gastroenterol Nutr* **11**: 83–88.
20. Minami J (1985) Helping mothers with Letdown. Oregon Areas Leaders' letter of La Leche League.
21. Yokoyama Y, Ueda T, Irahara M et al (1994) Releases of oxytocin and prolactin during breast massage and suckling in puerperal woman. *Eur J Obstet Gynaecol Reprod Biol* **53**: 17–20.
22. Bose CL, D'Ercole J, Lester AG et al (1981) Relactation by mothers of sick and preterm infants. *Pediatrics* **67**: 565–569.
23. Riordan J (1989) *A Practical Guide to Breastfeeding.* Boston: Jones & Bartlett, pp. 262–273.
24. De Carvalho M, Klaus MH, Merkatz RB (1982) Frequency of breast-feeding and serum bilirubin. *Am J Dis Child* **136**: 737–738.
25. MAIN Trial Collaborative Group (1994) Preparing for breastfeeding: treatment of inverted and non-protractile nipples in pregnancy. *Midwifery* **10**: 200–211.

Breast conditions

Keeping the mother's breasts healthy should always be one of the aims when caring for babies who are breastfed or receiving their mother's milk. The reality is that mothers with babies in a neonatal or paediatric unit are at more risk of breast problems than other mothers. This is not really surprising: the mother and her family are often under great stress; breastfeeding is commonly delayed for days or weeks; the mother may have to express 3-hourly irrespective of her other commitments; her baby may suffer setbacks; she may have to travel long distances to the hospital; and she may have other young children to care for. Even with continual support, problems are always likely to arise. To help a mother overcome any breast conditions quickly, a systematic approach is helpful:

◆ look for a cause and correct it
◆ give specific advice to the mother to prevent it happening again
◆ make other helpful suggestions
◆ treat as necessary
◆ monitor her progress.

4.1 THE NORMAL BREASTFEEDING EXPERIENCE

Mothers perceive the sensation of 'normal' breastfeeding differently. For some it is comfortable and pleasant from the beginning; others are surprised at how uncomfortable it feels and how strange the sensation is; and for a few mothers it is painful, particularly in the first few days. Tension can make this worse. The breasts are very delicate and maybe mothers should expect that breastfeeding will initially be different from anything else they have experienced. Even so, for many mothers it is a surprisingly pleasurable experience; for some it is even sensual. Any discomfort experienced by mothers in the first few days gradually disappears as time passes and breastfeeding is established. For others the discomfort remains without any reason being found – these mothers need a great deal of support, understanding and encouragement.

4.2 INITIAL OR PHYSIOLOGICAL FULLNESS OF THE BREAST

Fullness of the breast in the first few days after delivery is physiologically normal, and commonly occurs between 24 hours and 72 hours after delivery. It can be relatively mild and pass almost unnoticed, or severe and accompanied by pain and discomfort. This fullness is caused not only by the volume of milk increasing over a comparatively short time, but also by the venous system adjusting to hormonal changes. It should settle within 24–48 hours. A mother may experience noticeable fullness for at least the first 2–3 weeks, after which her breasts begin to feel softer, even before a feed.

All mothers, whether they breastfeed or bottle-feed, will experience some degree of initial fullness.[1] Reassure mothers who are bottle-feeding using a formula milk that, provided they do not stimulate their breasts or remove the breastmilk, the discomfort will pass. A firm, well-fitting brassière may help at this time.

The second or third day after delivery is commonly a time when a mother may feel tearful and emotional. If the baby is in a neonatal or paediatric unit, or has anything wrong with him, the mother's emotions may be even more labile. It is important, therefore, that she avoids preventable breast conditions, which may not only interfere with her ability to feed her baby, but also add to her general discomfort at this time.

Although there is no 'cure' for physiological fullness, it is self-limiting. Some of the practical advice below may help relieve some of the discomfort. It is important to tell a mother in advance about the breast fullness she may experience in the first few days after delivery, for then it will not worry her and she will know how to cope with it. Practical advice should include some or all of the following:

1. If the baby is term and able to feed without any problem, feeding him whenever he is hungry ('demand' feeding) will relieve the fullness created by the milk. This is a situation where a mother who is beginning to feel full can also try to wake her baby, even if he is sleepy, and encourage him to feed. At this stage, demand feeding is something that works both ways! The feeds should not be timed in length.
2. If expression of milk is necessary, it should be done regu-larly, at least 3-hourly. There should be no long intervals between expressions. Long periods between expressions or breastfeeding will only increase breast fullness and may cause pathological engorgement to occur at the same time. Advise the mother, if she is uncomfortable in the night, to express at that time or her breasts will feel much fuller in the morning.

3. If breast fullness is very uncomfortable, relief may be provided in the following ways:
   - ◆ bathing the breasts in warm or hot water in a bowl, bath or shower, and expressing enough milk for the breasts to be comfortable, or allowing any milk to drain naturally
   - ◆ covering the breasts with a warm or hot towel, gently massaging them, and then hand-expressing.
4. Use clean, washed cabbage leaves (smooth, dark-green leaves) to place around the breasts, making sure a hole is left for the nipple.[2,3] This is very comforting if the leaves have just come from a refrigerator. Support the leaves inside a brassière. It is thought that a substance in the leaves reduces oedema and improves milk flow. This is useful for physiological fullness, engorgement, and for mastitis – and is guaranteed to bring a smile to the afflicted at a difficult time! Prolonged use of the leaves is believed to reduce milk flow,[2] therefore the leaves should not be used for longer than is necessary to relieve the symptoms.
5. Take a mild analgesic for pain if necessary.

Reassure the mother that breast fullness is normal in the first few days and will last a short time only. If the nipples become flattened because of breast fullness, expression of a little milk by hand or with a hand pump before feeding will draw out the nipple, and soften the breast sufficiently to aid the baby to suckle. With physiological fullness the milk should flow without difficulty.

4.3 NIPPLES

A new baby has no preconceived idea of nipple or breast shape. At the time of delivery, babies who are born at term and who are healthy have no apparent difficulty in finding the breast and breastfeeding with the mother lying on her back – which does not enhance the shape of her nipple, areola or breast. Babies are driven by instinct to seek their mother's milk; the nipple just happens to be an important anatomical feature which when stimulated sets off milk production and milk flow – as the lactiferous sinuses that the baby must reach are rarely in the nipple itself, the baby has to take in a substantial amount of breast tissue to breastfeed effectively. Therefore, it should not be assumed because a mother has a nipple shape commonly perceived as causing problems, that it will actually do so. If the nipple and areola tissue is soft it will conform to the shape of the baby's mouth, so it is often not the nipple shape which is at fault for attachment failing to take place, but rather the position the baby is in.

There are many nipple shapes and sizes, and for the majority of babies they cause no real problems. However, some nipple shapes may create a challenge to babies needing special care; these include nipples that are long, large, flat or inverted. In some cases it is a matter of finding less conventional positions for the baby to feed in, and having patience until a small baby grows bigger.

4.3.1 Inverted and flat nipples

If inverted or flat nipples have been observed in the antenatal period (Figs 4.1 and 4.2) it does not mean a baby will have difficulty breastfeeding. After delivery the mother's areola and nipple area may show more protractility or elasticity than before or during pregnancy. Therefore, it is important to assess a breastfeed as soon as is practical after delivery to see if the shape of the mother's nipple is still likely to create a difficulty with feeding. After breastfeeding the nipple may be quite drawn out and prominent for a while. It is important to emphasize to the mother that the baby should be breastfeeding and not nipple feeding. Therefore, it is the **attachment** at the breast and the **positioning**, which is of crucial importance to the baby's success at breastfeeding.

Practically, an inverted nipple may show characteristics that do make it a challenge to any baby, not just those who require special care. Some inverted nipples can be easily pulled out, even though they then pop back into the areola; others disappear further (retract) into the areola when touched – these are 'tethered'. To quickly find out what type the mother has, get her to put her thumb and first finger on either side of the areola, with the nipple in between. Without moving the position of

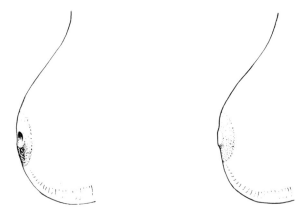

Figure 4.1 An inverted nipple.   **Figure 4.2** A flat nipple.

her thumb and forefinger, she should first of all gently push her forefinger into the areola tissue and release, and then push her thumb into the areola tissue and release. Using a rocking movement, she should repeat this several times. If the nipple is untethered it will pop out; if not, it will sink further into the areola and no amount of coaxing will make it emerge. It is the tethered nipple that creates most difficulty for attachment, and for which leaning positions are most useful in the first few days.

How to overcome most inverted or flat nipples

◆ Ensure the area around the nipple and areola is soft prior to breastfeeding.

◆ Stimulation of the nipples to make them as erect as possible may help with both nipple shapes. Gently rolling and pulling the nipple out, prior to breastfeeding, can achieve this.

◆ Use a breast reliever or a breast pump to soften the nipple, and encourage the nipple to become more prominent.

◆ Hand-express some milk into the baby's mouth to get him interested in the breast.

◆ Position the baby for feeding at the breast in such a way that attachment is made as easy as possible. Any position in which the breast is able to 'fall' into the baby's mouth may help for the first few breastfeeds; for example, having the baby lying on his mother's lap so that she can lean over with her breast falling into the baby's mouth; or the baby on a table, on the floor or on the bed with the mother leaning over him.

◆ Just before attachment, when the breast is 'falling' into the baby's mouth the mother should very gently press the underside of her breast with the edge of her first finger as close as she can to the areola without interfering with the baby's attachment. This makes an untethered inverted nipple pop out and may make attachment a little easier.

◆ Attach the baby to the breast, with his bottom lip on the underside of the areola aimed as far away from the junction of the nipple and areola as possible. His top lip or his nose should be in line with the nipple. Make sure his mouth is open as widely as possible (Fig. 4.3) prior to attachment. Bring him quickly to the breast once this occurs.

◆ Let the mother and baby spend a day in bed together, where the baby can have as much skin and breast contact as possible.

◆ A 10 mL or 20 mL syringe can also be used to help draw the nipple out just before a feed (Fig. 4.4).[4,5] The size of the syringe will depend upon the width of the nipple. Before doing this it should be established whether the nipple is tethered or untethered. If the nipple can be pulled out, the syringe will probably be helpful.

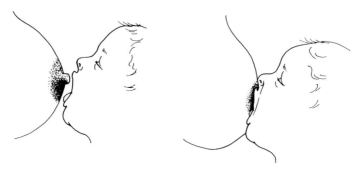

Figure 4.3 Attachment of a baby at the breast.

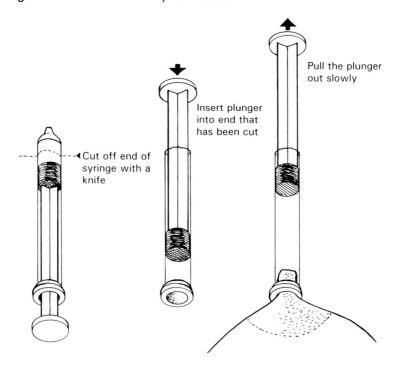

Figure 4.4 The syringe method of treating inverted nipples.

To prepare the syringe:

1. Cut approximately 3 cm off the nozzle end.
2. Remove the plunger and insert it into the cut end.
3. Place the smooth end of the syringe barrel over the nipple.
4. Pull the plunger **one-third** of the way out of the barrel. Be very gentle. Maintain the pressure applied.

5. The nipple should be drawn into the barrel.
6. Do not pull the plunger all the way out of the barrel: this makes it more difficult to remove the syringe without hurting the nipple.
7. To remove the syringe from the breast, push the plunger in, to release the suction.

This treatment can be used for a few seconds, just before attachment to the breast. However, if any pain is felt during the process, it is important to gently push the plunger in and release the suction created. This will prevent any damage occurring to the nipple or the areola. Damage is more likely to occur if the nipple is tethered by short ducts from the lactiferous sinuses to the nipple surface. No device, whether homemade or commercially designed to treat inverted nipples, should be left in place for any longer than is necessary to draw the nipple out (a few seconds in most cases). If the baby appears to be having extreme difficulties with attachment, it may be necessary for the mother to express her milk for the first 1–2 weeks and feed the baby by cup, while he is learning to breastfeed and the mother experiments with different positions.

Using breast shells or stretching exercises (Hoffman's exercises) in the antenatal period have not been found to be useful.[6,7] However, if mothers wish to try the exercises, as long as they are gentle they will not do any harm. Breast shells may put pressure on the milk ducts if the brassière is not slightly bigger than normal to accommodate the shell and the breast. Do not make negative comments to the mother about her nipple shape.

4.3.2 Long and large nipples

Preterm and small-for-dates babies have shallow mouths; in other words, if a mother has a long or a large nipple, the baby does not have enough room in his mouth for the nipple and for any breast tissue as well. This can lead to the mother developing sore nipples, and a frustrated baby, because he cannot reach the lactiferous sinuses, and the nipple may make him gag. Babies grow very quickly, and their mouths lengthen, so it may be necessary to wait a few days before breastfeeding is possible. The mother's nipples will remain the same. During this time the mother may express her milk and feed her baby by cup, but she should be encouraged to have as much skin contact with her new baby as possible.

How to overcome long nipples

◆ Do not stimulate the nipple; this only makes it longer or more fibrous if it is already large.
◆ Lightly wrap the baby so that his arms are secured and he cannot touch the breasts.

◆ Try a less conventional position, with the mother either lying on her back or leaning back in a chair so that her nipples are not so prominent; the baby can be positioned across her chest.

4.4 SORE AND CRACKED NIPPLES

These are best avoided! The majority of sore and cracked nipples are the result of incorrect positioning and attachment of the baby at the breast. It is therefore essential to ensure that all mothers are taught about attachment and positioning, and the importance of being able to maintain the position for the duration of the feed. In this way mothers should avoid this cause of damage to their breasts.

It is also essential not to assume that poor attachment and positioning are the *only* causes of sore and cracked nipples. To exclude other causes, a number of questions should be asked and the breast visually examined. If the information the mother gives you makes you think the problem may be poor attachment and positioning, then it is vital that you watch a feed and make corrections if they are necessary. If the mother's answers make you think there may be another cause for her discomfort, give her as much information and help to overcome the problem as possible, **but** also watch her breastfeed if you can, to make sure that poor attachment and positioning are not adding to her problems. Some mothers may have more than one problem causing soreness or cracked nipples. The following questions will help to diagnose what the problem or problems may be.

To find the cause of sore and cracked nipples, ask the mother:

◆ When does she feel the pain?
  – At the beginning of the feed? Does it get less or stay the same?
  – After a few minutes? Does it increase as the feed continues?
  – Before the feed begins?
  – After the feed?
  – All the time through a feed and at other times as well?
◆ Where does she feel the pain?
  – At her nipple tip?
  – In the nipple?
  – Inside her breast?
  – Somewhere else?
  – On the surface of the nipple and areola?
◆ What does the pain/sensation/discomfort feel like?
  – Excruciating?
  – Burning?
  – Like a bee-sting inside the breast, or like red-hot needles pushed into the breast?

– Stinging?
– Like a power shower behind the nipple?
– Dull, deep ache?
– Itchy?
◆ Is the pain or discomfort in one or both breasts?
– In one breast at the time of feeding?
– In both breasts at the time of feeding?
– In both breasts not associated with feeding?

Ask the mother what her nipple, areola or breast look like.
Observe the breast:

◆ Is the nipple discoloured? Is it red, pink or white?
◆ Is there an obvious crack anywhere?
◆ Is there any bleeding or discharge?
◆ What does the skin look like? Is it flaky or papery?

4.4.1 Common conditions causing sore nipples and breasts

Mothers may describe the following conditions in many different ways.
The notes after each condition use the most commonly heard descriptions,
but are by no means the only terms used. Pain is very subjective: 'discomfort' to one mother may be 'acute pain' to another. If a mother complains
about 'pain', 'discomfort' or abnormal 'sensations' anywhere in or on her
breast, always take her seriously and investigate further. Try not to jump to
conclusions about what may be wrong. Sometimes discomfort may be felt
in the whole breast and a mother will find it difficult to pinpoint exactly
where she feels the discomfort or pain. Therefore some of the common
reasons for general breast pain are also included in the following list.

Poor attachment

Pain is acute at the beginning of the feed, usually diminishing as the
feed continues. The pain is felt at the tip of the nipple or over the whole
skin of the nipple and areola. It is not a deep pain. It is sometimes
described as a stinging pain or as if the 'skin is burning or on fire'. The
pain is usually exquisite in its initial intensity. It is experienced in the
breast the baby is feeding from.

The nipple may be inflamed or mildly pink, but sometimes there is
little to be seen. The nipple may appear to be misshapen after the feed.

Thrush (candidiasis)

Pain caused by thrush (infection with *Candida albicans*) gradually
increases after the feed begins and often continues well after the feed

finishes – sometimes for as much as an hour. It is described in a number of ways. If thrush is on the surface of the skin only, there may be intense pain and sometimes itchiness in the nipple; if thrush has gone into the milk ducts, the pain may be described as a stabbing or an intense burning pain. It is also described as being like 'red-hot needles' stabbed into the breast or a 'bee-sting' inside the breast. The pain can be felt in the whole nipple or deep within the breast. It is experienced in the breast the baby is feeding from. The pain may suddenly start after some days or weeks of pain-free breastfeeding, or it may be present from the time of the birth.

There may be nothing to see on the nipple and areola. Sometimes the areola may look pink, or red and papery, there may be slight swelling, and the skin may look flaky. On brown or black skin, the areola and nipple may be discoloured and appear pale or pink. The mother may crave sweet foods.

Check the baby for signs of thrush.

Nipple blanching and Raynaud's phenomenon

Pain is acute after the feed. It may be a throbbing and burning intense pain felt in the nipple and areola as the blood supply returns. It is experienced in the breast the baby is feeding from. Initially after the feed the nipple and part of the areola are completely white. As the blood supply returns the nipple and areola become very red; this is when the pain is at its most intense.

Forceful let-down

Pain develops as the feed progresses. It is experienced 'inside' or near the areola area. It may feel like a 'power shower' inside the breast, behind the areola, or an uncomfortable and painful 'tingling' sensation. The symptoms may sound similar to those of thrush, except that the pain is felt in *both* breasts at the same time during feeding. However, the pain may be more acute in the breast that the baby is feeding from compared with the other breast.

Eczema, dermatitis or allergy

This may cause a persistent irritation of the nipple and areola, and include the whole breast. At the time of breastfeeding, the skin of the nipple and areola may sting and feel itchy. The skin may look flaky and dry; the nipple and areola may look raw, inflamed or pink. It is felt on the surface of both breasts all the time, and more acutely at the time of feeding on each breast (at the time of feeding).

Prolactin surge

This is often experienced at night and is not apparently associated with the time of feeding. Some mothers will describe a deep ache in both breasts at the same time, others will describe it as a pain which is deep in the breasts, which will not go away.

Heavy breasts

In some mothers, heavy breasts may be the cause of a deep ache in both breasts at the same time and in their back, during the day and night and between feeds.

4.4.2 Cracks on the nipple

In addition to soreness a mother may have a visible crack or cracks on her nipple or areola. These will almost certainly cause her pain, particularly at the beginning of a feed. Where the cracks are can give a clue as to the cause:

At the tip of the nipple

A crack on the tip of the nipple can be caused by:

◆ Poor attachment. Only the nipple is in the baby's mouth. The tongue is not far enough forward, so there is active friction from the front part of the tongue on the tip of the nipple, causing a crack or generalized raw area. No other damage can be seen. After the feed the nipple may appear 'squashed', with a prominent line along the tip **before** the crack appears.

◆ Tongue tie (ankyloglossia) causes similar damage to the tip of the mother's nipple as poor attachment, and for the same reason. The tongue is too far back in the mouth and therefore friction of the tongue damages the skin of the tip or sides of the nipple. There may also be some degree of 'nipple biting' because the baby cannot get his tongue under the nipple and out over the bottom gums and jaw, so the nipple is compressed between the upper and lower gums, causing rawness around the sides of the nipple.

Around the base of the nipple

Cracks around the base of the nipple at the junction with the areola can be caused by:

◆ Poor attachment and positioning. If a baby is unable to maintain attachment at the breast because his position changes slightly, there may be a degree of tension in the breast tissue in the baby's mouth. Continued suckling causes some movement of the tissue in and out of the baby's mouth, and the area around the junction of the nipple and areola is stretched to a point where the skin is damaged and cracks.

◆ The funnel used by a mother expressing her milk by pump may be too large for her nipple and areola. There may be excessive movement of the breast tissue in and out of the funnel, causing tension at the junction between the nipple and areola. This results in a fine crack at this sensitive point.

At the tip and around the base

Cracks at the tip and around the base of the nipple may be caused by poor attachment and positioning. If the mouth is not widely opened for correct attachment, or the nipple is aimed at the centre of the mouth, the nipple and areola will not go far enough into the baby's mouth for him to suckle effectively. There may be excessive movement of the breast tissue in and out of the mouth compounded by the tongue being too far back in the mouth, or the tip of the nipple moving against the roof of the baby's mouth. This will cause damage to the tip and the base or sides of the nipple.

In addition to cracks on the nipple where there is excessive movement of the breast tissue, either from poor attachment and positioning or from movement in a funnel or Flexi-shield, there may also be visible oedema of the areola.

Other causes

In addition to the situations mentioned above, sore and cracked nipples may be caused, or made worse, by:

◆ The baby licking or biting the nipple.
◆ The baby being pulled off the breast when attached, without the seal around the breast being broken first.
◆ Any dryness of the nipple and areola caused by eczema, dermatitis or an allergic reaction can increase the risk of the nipples becoming cracked, especially if there is also poor attachment and positioning.
◆ Any infection of the nipple and areola affecting the skin makes it more susceptible to cracking, particularly if the skin is slightly oedematous as well.
◆ Thrush, which may prevent a crack from healing properly.

There is no evidence to suggest that fair-skinned mothers are any more likely to suffer sore or cracked nipples than any other mothers.

4.4.3 What to do about sore and cracked nipples

First of all, look for the cause of the soreness or nipple damage. This involves:

◆ asking the mother questions that help to diagnose the problem
◆ examining the mother's breasts and examining her baby for signs of thrush or tongue tie
◆ observing the mother breastfeeding.

Then treat the mother and give general advice to help prevent recurrence of the problem.
Some advice is general to many conditions.

Sore nipples without cracks

At the time of feeding

◆ Begin the milk flow before putting the baby to the breast, i.e. hand-express a little milk on to the nipple.
◆ A warm, damp flannel on the breast can help to encourage the milk to flow.
◆ Some mothers find it helpful to begin the feed on the unaffected or less sore side first. The vigorous suckling action that may be experienced at the start of a feed will have become gentler when the baby is attached to the sore breast.
◆ Attach and position the baby correctly. If pain continues, reposition the baby and reattach him. Sometimes a completely different position may be helpful.
◆ Some mothers may find that giving the baby 10–15 mL of breast-milk by cup before the feed begins helps to reduce the initial vigour of the baby's suck, particularly if he is very hungry.
◆ A nipple shield is seldom of any use in this situation. If one is used, the mother should be aware this is **a temporary solution only**. Nipple shields may be a cause of sore or cracked nipples if they do not fit exactly, because they cause stress to the delicate area at the junction of the nipple and areola.

Between feeds or expressing

◆ Remove brassière and breast pads until the nipples are healed. If the mother finds it uncomfortable without a brassière, suggest she wears either a cotton stretch cropped top (Fig. 4.5) or supports her breasts with a cotton scarf loosely tied around her body (Fig. 4.6).
◆ Some mothers may find that expressing a little milk on to the nipple and smoothing it around the sore area helps the healing process, although there is little research to show that this works.

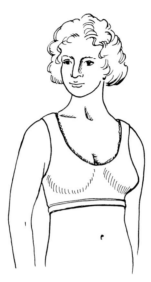

Figure 4.5 A comfortable support for the breasts – a cropped top.

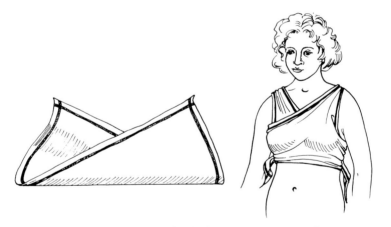

Figure 4.6 A comfortable support for the breasts – a cotton scarf.

◆ Keep the breasts exposed to the air or under loose clothing, preferably made of a natural fibre such as cotton.

No other treatment is usually necessary.

Nipples that are cracked and sore

Follow the above advice, paying particular attention to the correct attachment and positioning of the baby. Reassure the mother that once this is done, the cracks, although painful, will usually heal very quickly – particularly if they are caused by mechanical damage.

In addition:

◆ If the cracks in the nipple make it too painful to feed, use the unaffected side only (if possible).

◆ If the mother does not feed from the affected side, she should express her milk. This should be done at least every 3 hours to avoid engorgement. Hand-expression is the preferred method because hand and mechanical pumps can make cracks worse. If the mother still wants to express with a mechanical pump, she should use the lowest setting and stop using it if the discomfort becomes more acute. The milk expressed is safe to give to the baby, unless it is heavily contaminated with blood (which may cause the baby to vomit).

◆ If both the nipples are painful, gently hand-express to start the milk flow, and then attach the baby at the breast – making absolutely sure the mother's nipple is opposite the baby's nose or upper lip at the time of attachment.

◆ There is some anecdotal evidence that, for sore nipples, geranium leaves give 'instant relief if the furry side is placed on the nipple'.[8]

◆ Mothers should avoid, as far as possible, creams, ointments or sprays that claim to relieve nipple soreness. Most do not work, although if the mother has found something that helps her, unless there are known contraindications she should continue to use it.

◆ In recent years, a treatment known as **moist wound healing** has become popular for cracked nipples.[9] It uses ultrarefined lanolin which has had all the allergens removed. Only a very small amount is applied to the crack. It does not have to be washed off for feeding. Some women find their sore and cracked nipples heal very quickly. In some hospitals paraffin gauze sheet dressings are used instead, also with positive results.[10]

If a mother finds the pain from a sore or cracked nipple seriously interferes with breastfeeding, she can express her breastmilk and rest her breasts for one or more feeds. She can give her milk to her baby by cup, or by gastric tube if this is considered appropriate. Once her breasts feel more comfortable she can resume breastfeeding.

Advice for specific conditions

In some cases, treatment is specific to the condition diagnosed.

Poor attachment

◆ Check the baby's attachment.
◆ If either attachment or positioning are not correct, ask the mother to stop feeding.

- To remove the baby from the breast, the mother should slide her little finger into the baby's mouth. This breaks the seal he has made with his lips around the areola and breast tissue.
- Help the mother position and reattach her baby. She may still feel discomfort when he first suckles, but the pain should be less if the breast tissue is in the right place inside his mouth.
- There is no need to rest the breast.

Thrush (candidiasis)

- Tell the mother to wash her hands well before she breastfeeds.
- Check in the baby's mouth. Look for white patches, on the tongue, roof of the mouth, sides of the mouth. Check his bottom; is it red, spotty and sore-looking, and slow to get better? Sometimes the baby shows no signs at all but still has thrush. Is he unhappy at the breast?
- Treatment for the mother:[11,12] treat skin thrush with **Daktarin** cream (miconazole). Apply a small amount to the nipple, *after* each feed. Treat thrush inside the breast with **nystatin tablets,** 500 000 units 6-hourly for 14 days, or **fluconazole capsules,** 150 mg for the first dose, then 50 mg twice a day for 10 days.[13]
- Treatment for the baby: give **Daktarim** (miconzole) oral gel or **nystatin** drops four times a day, *after* feeds. Treat the baby even if he shows no signs of thrush. The mother should see her own doctor before starting these drugs. She should also tell the staff of the neonatal or paediatric unit that she has thrush. Once treatment begins, an improvement should be felt within a few days.
- If the baby is diagnosed as having thrush, the mother may need to use Daktarin (miconazole) cream prophylactically.
- Heat is very effective at killing the spores that cause thrush. Tell the mother to wash her underwear, sheets, towels and clothes in a washing machine, using the hottest wash. Ironing also kills the fungal spores.
- Ask the mother if she or the baby has been on antibiotics recently. Thrush commonly occurs following a course of antibiotics.
- Avoid using dummies, they are a common source of thrush in babies.
- Advise the mother to eat yoghurt containing active *Lactobacillus acidophilus.* This can change the nature of the bacteria in the mother's gut, which can help to limit fungal growth. Breastfeeding the baby encourages the growth of specific gut flora such as lactobacilli, which also limit fungal growth – so it is important not to stop breastfeeding if thrush is diagnosed. Acidophilus capsules (including vegan formulas) can be bought from health-food shops.

Nipple blanching and Raynaud's phenomenon

Nipple blanching and Raynaud's phenomenon can be caused by some drug therapies such as theophylline; by smoking, as nicotine causes vasoconstriction; caffeine; the cold; and by the baby 'biting' the nipple.[14]

◆ Seek advice on any drugs that may cause this condition. Cut down or stop smoking and reduce caffeine intake.
◆ Wear warm clothing. A warm compress placed over the areola before feeding may help.
◆ Some mothers find adding fish oil to their diet helps, others find evening primrose oil works well.
◆ Sometimes drinking tea will help!
◆ In very severe cases the drug **nifedipine** has been shown to help.[13] A doctor should be consulted if the problem is severe.

Forceful let-down

Reassure the mother that this will gradually subside.

Eczema, dermatitis or allergy

◆ Ask the mother if she has changed her washing powder, soap or body lotion recently or whether she has started to eat something different from her normal diet. These are common causes of eczema or dermatitis suddenly appearing.
◆ Plastic-backed breast pads or nipple shields may irritate the skin of some mothers and should be avoided if they are the cause.
◆ Advise the mother not to use soap or perfumed creams on her breasts.

Heavy breasts

A well-fitting, supportive brassière may help to alleviate the problem of heavy breasts during the day. Wearing a brassière at night as well may help, as long as it is not restrictive.

Sore and cracked nipples, if not treated, are a possible entry point for more serious infection, which may cause infective mastitis.

4.5 PATHOLOGICAL ENGORGEMENT

Pathological engorgement should not happen. It occurs when milk is not regularly removed from the breast by either breastfeeding or by expression. Milk is allowed to build up, causing increasing distension of the whole breast. It can happen at any time during lactation, particularly in the early days of breastfeeding, and like fullness, it usually affects both breasts.

This kind of engorgement may also be caused by inefficient drainage of all or some of the functioning lobes of the breast during a feed.

This results from incorrect attachment and positioning of the baby. Poor attachment may lead to excess stimulation of the nipple by the tongue, resulting in increased milk production adding to the engorgement.

Pathologically engorged breasts may look shiny, red and oedematous, and the mother may complain that they feel 'tight' and painful. The nipple is often flattened, making attachment difficult to achieve, and the milk does not flow easily. The following suggestions can be used to relieve this situation:

◆ Remove some milk by hand or pump to soften the breast sufficiently either to breastfeed or to express. Use a 'syringe' type of cylinder pump, or a 'bicycle horn' type pump. Be very gentle. Remember to discard the milk expressed with this type of pump.
◆ The mother can bathe her breasts in a shower or bath to encourage the milk to drain.
◆ Lean over a sink or basin of warm water and 'dunk' the breasts in the water. This will also encourage milk flow.
◆ Stimulate the oxytocin reflex by back, breast and nipple massage.
◆ The partner can help suck some of the milk from the breast.
◆ **Areolar massage** can be used. This is best done initially by a second person.
  - The thumbs should be placed on either side of the areola over the area of the lactiferous sinuses.
  - Using firm rolling movements the thumbs should move from the outside of the areola margin (or where the mother has felt the lactiferous sinuses) towards the nipple.
  - This rolling movement should be done all around the areola.
  - It may take 5–10 minutes before the milk begins to flow.
  - Usually the milk begins to flow slowly and as the areolar area becomes softer the milk flow is faster.
  - Once the areola and nipple are soft enough for the mother to breastfeed her baby or express her milk, the massage can stop.
◆ Cabbage leaves may help relieve some of the discomfort.
◆ Line a large pudding basin with ice, or with frozen peas, which have been put into a large plastic bag (they can then be shaped more easily than in the bought packaging). Cover the ice with a tea towel. Lean over the basin and let the breast fall into it. This will help reduce oedema; do this after feeding.

Pathological engorgement can be avoided by using the advice already given for initial or physiological fullness. If engorgement continually happens, the mother's milk supply will begin to diminish due to the action of the feedback inhibitor of lactation. The best way to prevent pathological engorgement is to make sure a mother feeds her baby or expresses her milk regularly, without long intervals overnight.

4.6 BLOCKED DUCTS, LOBES, MASTITIS AND BREAST ABSCESS

All of these are best avoided. The advice contained already in this chapter and in Chapter 2 (positioning and attachment) will certainly help to prevent these conditions.

4.6.1 Blocked ducts and lobes

If any small ducts in the nipple or leading into the lactiferous sinuses become blocked and milk cannot drain, lobes can very quickly become uncomfortably full of milk. It is essential, therefore, to keep the nipples healthy and handle the breast correctly.

The following situations may cause blocked ducts and subsequently lead to full lobes:

◆ incorrect attachment or positioning
◆ irregular breastfeeding or expression
◆ incorrect hand-expression or rough handling of the breasts, causing trauma to the nipples or ducts
◆ sore, cracked nipples, which may cause swelling to occur in or around the tiny ducts leading from the lactiferous sinuses to the surface of the nipple
◆ compression from the fingers holding the breast during a feed – particularly the 'scissor' hold (Fig. 4.7)
◆ a brassière or clothing that is not loose enough during feeding, expression or between feeds, and causes continual pressure on any part of the breast

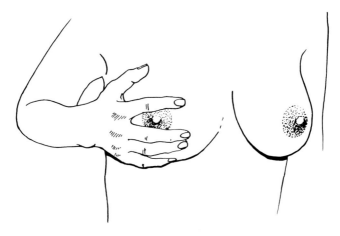

Figure 4.7 The 'scissor' hold.

◆ large breasts which are not drained effectively during feeding or expression
◆ a weakness in any part of the breast from a previous injury – even one occurring in childhood, such as being hit in the breast, or being kicked by a horse (this can be one possible cause of recurrent mastitis in the same place).

Signs of blocked ducts and lobes

◆ Unusual tenderness or hardness in one segment of the breast. The outline of any underlying lump often follows the margins of a lobe (more than one lobe may be affected if a duct in the nipple is blocked).
◆ A patch of red skin often appears over the hard, tender area.

Suggested management

Treatment is aimed at restoring the milk flow as soon as possible, otherwise mastitis will develop and, if this is not properly treated, an abscess may form. This can happen very quickly, within 24–48 hours. Advise the mother to continue breastfeeding. If she stops, the problem will become more acute. The suggested treatment is as follows:

1. Feed the baby whenever he is willing to suckle. Try to avoid long gaps between feeds, especially during the acute phase of the condition. This may mean expressing the breastmilk if the baby does not want to suckle regularly.

2. Assess the baby's attachment at the breast and improve this if necessary, so that all the lactiferous sinuses are drained efficiently. Leaning forward will help drain the breasts if they are heavy or pendulous. A small, rolled-up towel or flannel placed under the breast will help to enhance drainage of the lobes (Fig. 4.8). Make sure that the baby's position is stable and not likely to affect his correct attachment. Feed him from both breasts if possible.

3. Gently massage the affected part of the breast prior to expression, using the 'fingers' method of massage, or using the finger tips or a wide-toothed comb. Alternate the massage with expression until the breast is comfortable.

4. Express as much milk as possible by hand or pump. Where a mother is feeding a small or ill baby intermittently by breast, express any excess milk after a feed.

5. A bath or shower, or application of a warm flannel or towel to the affected breast prior to feeding will usually help the milk to flow.

6. Use another position to feed the baby.

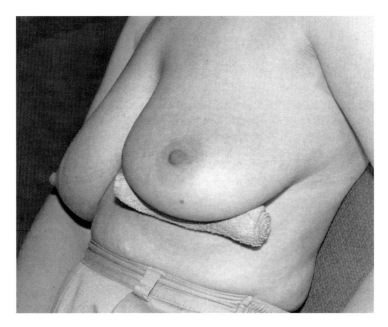

Figure 4.8 A small, rolled-up flannel placed under the breast to enhance drainage of the lobes.

7. Some mothers may find vigorous arm movements help, by encouraging the blood circulation.
8. Cabbage leaves may provide some relief.

Prevention

◆ Ensure correct positioning and attachment of the baby during a breastfeed.
◆ The baby should be fed regularly and on demand.
◆ If expressing, do so every 2–3 hours. Express overnight.
◆ Avoid tight clothing around the breast.
◆ If a baby has an eye infection, make sure it is cleaned prior to breastfeeding.
◆ Support a large or pendulous breast with a rolled-up flannel, as described in point 2 above.

4.6.2 White spot

Occasionally a mother may notice a small, white spot on the tip of her nipple, which cannot easily be removed. The 'spot' may be either a small calcium deposit or composed of fatty material, and forms a plug at the exit of one of the narrow ducts in the nipple. The mother may experience an intense localized pain in her nipple and within her areola, and have a tender area in her breast where the duct is blocked.

The white spot needs to be removed. This can be achieved by:

◆ the baby suckling (it is advisable to put the baby to this breast at the beginning of the feed as this is when his suckling is at its strongest)
◆ expression either by hand or pump (a pump may be more effective as it may have a stronger suction)
◆ using a clean fingernail or towel
◆ using a sterile needle to hook it out
◆ or the mother's partner may be able to suck it out.

There is usually immediate relief when the plug is removed, and the milk is again flowing. If it is not dealt with, it can go on to cause a blocked lobe and mastitis.

4.6.3 Mastitis

Mastitis will develop if a blocked duct is not treated promptly. In approximately 50% of cases it is non-infective,[15] and will respond to the treatment given in the above section. It is not necessary to give up breastfeeding, indeed this may make the condition worse. However, a baby may refuse his mother's milk because it tastes salty, due to increased sodium in the milk.[16] If this occurs it is very important to express the milk. The inflammation and pain that may accompany mastitis is caused by milk being forced out of the alveoli into the surrounding breast tissue. This causes a localized and acute inflammatory reaction to occur. It is sometimes difficult without culturing the milk to know if an infection is also present. In both infective or non-infective mastitis the initial treatment is exactly the same.

Signs of mastitis

The signs are:

◆ painful breasts
◆ a hot, red, firm swelling – often following the shape of one or two lobes
◆ there may be fever and flu-like symptoms, e.g. aching, lethargy
◆ the mother feels very unwell.

Suggested management

Continue breastfeeding!

1. Follow the suggestions already described for blocked lobes and ducts.

2. Start each feed from the affected side, if possible. Gently massage the breast before and during the feed, using the 'fingers' method, or with the fingertips or a comb.

3. Drainage of the milk is vital, no matter how it is achieved. If there is still discomfort after feeding, then expression with a pump or by hand is necessary. Hand-expression may be more comfortable.

4. Apply hot and/or cold compresses to the affected area between feeds, whichever is most comfortable.

5. Remember the cabbage leaves, especially if they are just taken out of a refrigerator – they may help soothe the breast.

6. Give analgesia to the mother, if required (e.g. **paracetamol**).

7. Anti-inflammatory drugs such as **ibuprofen** are becoming more commonly used to treat mastitis, particularly when it first begins. If there is no noticeable improvement after 24 hours, despite 3-hourly drainage of milk by breastfeeding or by expression, the mother should consult her doctor, midwife or health visitor.

8. If pain or inflammation continues despite following the advice so far given, a doctor must be consulted promptly. Antibiotics may be necessary. However, breastfeeding should be continued. Antibiotics may cause diarrhoea in the baby, who may then require more frequent feeding. This will usually help relieve the mastitis more quickly and will not harm the baby.

9. If the mother is feverish, make sure she does not become dehydrated.

10. Encourage the mother to rest, and to delegate the shopping, cooking and cleaning to someone else.

4.6.4 Breast abscess

A breast abscess, like mastitis, is commonly the result of a combination of poor milk removal from the breast and a bacterial infection. In an abscess, the infection localizes and pus forms inside a well-defined capsule. This may be situated near to the areola, or in the deeper tissue, as a result of unresolved mastitis or abrupt weaning.

Once the abscess has formed the pus must be drained. This needs to be done surgically,[16] either by incision or by ultrasound-guided aspiration. The mother will also need antibiotics. Although aspiration can be performed as an outpatient procedure, the mother is commonly admitted to a surgical ward for drainage of the abscess. If her baby is in a neonatal or paediatric hospital it may not be possible for her to have her baby admitted with her. In this case she should express her milk until she can resume breastfeeding. If the baby can be brought to her for feeds this will be very beneficial. It is essential that the surgical team are made aware that the mother is breastfeeding or expressing and that her baby is also in hospital.

If the mother has been expressing milk, she may already have some in the refrigerator; however, if she has been breastfeeding, she may need to express enough milk prior to surgical treatment for her baby's next feed.

The mother will need the help of a health professional with expertise in breastfeeding while she is in the surgical unit. She may need to borrow a breast pump, and may also need help with hand-expression, particularly for the affected breast. Although an abscess may result in a decrease in the mother's milk production on the affected side in **this** lactation, it should not affect her chances of breastfeeding again in the future.

The mother should be reassured that she *can* continue to breastfeed or express her milk.

Signs of breast abscess

The signs are:

◆ a very painful, well-defined swollen lump
◆ the skin over the lump may be reddened, hot and oedematous
◆ a generalized feeling of being unwell
◆ a fever may or may not be present; fever can occur very suddenly.

Suggested management following surgical drainage

1. The mother can continue feeding or expressing breastmilk from the **unaffected** breast either when she has come round from general anaesthesia (in the case of incision), or after aspiration under a local anaesthesia.

2. Breastfeeding or expression can be resumed on the **affected** side once the pain is sufficiently controlled. The mother may require analgesia.

3. Although there is little evidence to show that milk containing pus will harm a baby,[16] for babies in a neonatal unit who are already vulnerable it is probably safer to discard the milk from the **affected** side until it is clear of infective bacteria. This may mean sending the milk to the laboratory for analysis. However, milk from the **unaffected side can safely be given to the baby**. A mother is able to sustain her baby from one breast.

4. Milk from the **affected** breast should be expressed by hand. Expression needs to be done as gently as possible to avoid any further trauma to the tissues. Hand-expression is known to be bacteriologically safer than expression by pump.[17]

5. The mother may find she needs to use a different feeding position. Discuss alternative positions with her **before** surgical treatment.

She may need a skilled carer to help her with attaching her baby for the first few hours after treatment.

6. It is important to continue regular expression or encouraging the baby to suckle regularly on the affected side, so that the milk in the breast is regularly removed and the problem does not recur. However, milk production may be less than before, and in some cases where the abscess was very large, it may be difficult to increase production, from that breast.

7. The mother may require advice on relactation to increase milk production on the affected side.

Remember that **prevention is better than cure**! Treat any predisposing factor as it occurs.

4.7 BREASTFEEDING AND NIPPLE SHIELDS

Nipple shields (Fig. 4.9) **should not** be used without a very good reason. There is convincing evidence to suggest they can inhibit milk production, as stimulation of the nipple and breast is considerably reduced.[18,19] They are totally unsuitable for long-term use without specialist advice and, when they are used, they should be dispensed with as soon as possible.

Once a baby is used to feeding with a shield, it is extremely difficult to get him to breastfeed without it. The shield is used because a problem

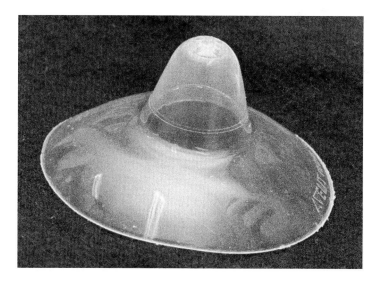

Figure 4.9 A nipple shield.

exists. It is important, therefore, before being tempted to use one, to assess the problem, and see if a solution can be found that avoids its use. Despite the short-term gains, using a nipple shield may prove to be much more troublesome and time-consuming in the long term. The fact that a baby is feeding 'well' with a shield does not mean the problem has been solved. Its use may adversely affect the mother's chances of establishing breastfeeding, unless considerable care is taken.

However, in spite of all the qualms one has about using nipple shields, it is something we should always keep in reserve – for the very rare occasions when it may make the difference between a stressed, tired mother, in the middle of the night, having a 'nervous breakdown' and giving breastfeeding up for good, or just trying one more time, because for whatever reason, her baby has spent the last 3 hours wanting to feed but absolutely refusing to attach to the breast. If you know absolutely everything possible has been done to help both the mother and baby … then using a shield may help overcome a very difficult and stressful period. But next day the whole situation may need careful thought to make sure whatever problem has led to the distress is dealt with in a sympathetic and positive way. For example, it might help to encourage the mother and baby to bathe together in a relaxed way so that the baby can, in his own time, find the breast and feed (see below).[20]

4.7.1 How to avoid the use of nipple shields

1. Teach mothers how to hand-express:
   – to avoid sore nipples
   – to start the milk flow at the beginning of the feed
   – to express directly into the baby's mouth.
2. Ensure the baby is positioned and attached correctly and appropriately for his size and gestation.
3. If the mother's nipples are flat or inverted, teach her to:
   – gently massage the nipples, to make them become more erect
   – use a hand pump or breast reliever prior to the feed, to draw the nipple out, or to soften the breast, if it is engorged
   – possibly use cold water or ice to make the nipples erect.
4. If the baby 'fights' at the breast:
   – Feed the baby expressed breastmilk by cup until he calms down.
   – Use the breastfeeding supplementer.
   – Avoid using a bottle teat, dummy or nipple shield. All of these may give a baby who is to be breastfed an inappropriate experience of sucking. Sucking on a finger is likely to be of a shorter duration than using a dummy or nipple shield, but this may also confuse a baby if it occurs frequently. All of these sucking devices may cause him to refuse to suckle correctly at the breast.

 – Arrange for the mother and baby to bathe together. They will need to be supervised. The water should be comfortably warm, without being hot. It should reach the mother's lower chest when she leans back against the bath. She should have her baby placed on her chest between her breasts so that he can easily reach the nipples and areola to feed. The carer with the mother and baby should gently pour water over the baby's back so that he remains warm. This may help the baby to 'rediscover' the breast.

If, after trying to overcome the problem, it is still thought necessary – by either the mother or the professional adviser – to use a nipple shield, make sure the mother is aware of the following points:

◆ Less suction will be felt than when the baby is suckling directly from the breast (the tip of the shield can be cut off to help alleviate this).
◆ The shield is only a temporary measure. It is not a permanent solution to the original problem.
◆ Continuous use of a shield may compromise the baby's weight gain. This is because decreased breast stimulation causes a reduction in the milk production, which leads to a diminished milk supply.
◆ If the mother wishes or insists on using a nipple shield when her baby leaves the hospital, make sure that she is followed up by the health visitor or the health professional who has been advising her in hospital or a breastfeeding counsellor. The baby will require regular weighing, either by returning to the hospital unit or to the local health centre.
◆ She must only use the thin silicone nipple shields. These come in two sizes. The smaller size frequently provides a better fit, though neither size is really satisfactory.

4.7.2 Situations in which a nipple shield may be appropriate

It has to be acknowledged that some mothers have used nipple shields for long periods without apparent difficulty,[21,22] but it must be emphasized that these mothers are in a minority. Most of them will have experienced difficulties which probably could have been avoided with skilled help. The use of a shield may be appropriate in cases of:

 ◆ a truly inverted, non-protractile nipple (if all else has consistently failed)
 ◆ a baby with a cleft lip and/or palate, if his mother does not have protractile nipples (however, this should be used as a last resort, because this mother may not get sufficient breast stimulation without a shield and will receive even less with one)

◆ too much milk; using a nipple shield will reduce the nipple stimulation and may result in less milk being produced

◆ where a mother is giving her baby expressed breastmilk by bottle, but wants to breastfeed occasionally; she may want to use a nipple shield as the baby is used to the greater stimulus of a teat

◆ extremely traumatized nipples, where a mother does not wish to rest and express her breasts. In this case, correct advice on how to position and attach the baby is of paramount importance, as well as advice on how to deal with her sore nipples. The nipple shield should be discontinued as soon as possible because it will only add to her problems, and may actually be made worse by any movement in and out of the shield, if it does not fit exactly.

Never use a nipple shield when a baby, term or preterm, is first learning to breastfeed (i.e. in the first few days after delivery, or after several days or weeks if the baby is unable to breastfeed at birth) – it is not a substitute for teaching correct positioning or attachment.

4.7.3 How to use nipple shields

◆ Only use the thin silicone nipple shields (use the smaller size initially).
◆ Always hand-express a little milk into the nipple shield prior to the feed.
◆ Make sure the shield fits the mother's nipple as closely as possible.
◆ At the end of the feed, make sure there is evidence of milk in the shield.

4.7.4 How to wean a baby off the shield

There is no right or wrong way to wean a baby off a nipple shield. The method depends upon the baby and, to a great extent, the determination of the mother – and the support and help of the professional staff. It is also dependent on what the original problem was, the strategy adopted to solve it, and how often the shield has been and is being used.

When the shield has been used only once or twice:

1. Make sure the baby is positioned and attached at the breast correctly.
2. Hand-express some milk on to the nipple.
3. Ensure the baby opens his mouth widely before he latches on to the nipple and areola.
4. Hand-expressing directly into the baby's mouth initially may help.
5. If the baby is a healthy, term, 'well-padded' baby, do not even consider using the nipple shield again – even if the baby complains

bitterly! If the shield is given, the situation will just become more difficult and traumatic to correct. It is better to have a short period of agitation than risk the mother's milk supply long-term. When the baby is hungry enough, he will take the breast!

If the baby continues to refuse the breast:

6. Advise the mother to take her baby to bed with her for 24 hours, so that he has plenty of opportunity to feed from the breast whenever he is hungry or thirsty.
7. Encourage as much skin-to-skin contact as possible, especially prior to feed times.

Where the shield has been used for 1–2 days or longer, or where it has been used with a small or underweight baby, the method may be less straightforward:

1. If the mother and baby are relaxed at the beginning of the feed, try using the above methods first. If, however, after 5–10 minutes there is no success, use the nipple shield.
2. Alternatively use the shield for a fraction of the feed. For example, if a feed normally takes 15 minutes, use the shield for 5 minutes. Then try to attach the baby at the breast when the milk is flowing well and the breast tissue soft.
3. As already suggested, encourage the mother to have a day in bed with her baby and encourage skin-to-skin contact as often as possible.
4. Use the breastfeeding supplementer.
5. Fill a syringe with expressed breastmilk, and squeeze a little milk on to the nipple or areola just before the baby is offered the breast. This is useful when the mother is very tense and her milk is not flowing easily.

REFERENCES

1. Parazzini F, Zanaboni F, Liberati A et al (1989) Breast symptoms in women who are not breastfeeding. In: *Effective Care in Pregnancy and Childbirth.* Enkin M, Keirse M, Chalmers I (eds). Oxford: Oxford University Press, pp. 1390–1403.
2. Rosier W (1989) Cool cabbage compresses. *Breastfeeding Rev* **12**: 28.
3. Nikodem VC, Danziger D, Gebka N et al (1993) Do cabbage leaves prevent breast engorgement? A randomised, controlled study. *Birth* **20**: 61–64.
4. WHO/UNICEF (1993) *Breastfeeding Counselling: A Training Course Secretariat,* Division of Diarrhoeal and Acute Respiratory Disease Control, Session 14. Geneva: WHO, pp. 194–195.
5. Kesaree N, Banapurnath CR, Banapurnath S et al (1993) Treatment of inverted nipples using a disposable syringe. *J Hum Lact* **9**: 27–29.

6. Alexander JM, Grant AM, Campbell MJ (1992) Randomised controlled trial of breast shells and Hoffman's exercises for inverted and non-protractile nipples. *BMJ* **304**: 1030–1032.

7. MAIN Trial Collaborative Group (1994) Preparing for breastfeeding: treatment of inverted and non-protractile nipples in pregnancy. *Midwifery* **10**: 200–211.

8. Lloyd J (1992) Now geraniums? *Aust Lactation Consult Assoc News* **3**: 3–4.

9. Huml S (1999) Sore nipples. A new look at an old problem through the eyes of a dermatologist. *Pract Midwife* **2**: 28–31.

10. Inch S, Fisher C (2000) Breastfeeding: early problems. *Pract Midwife* **3**: 12–15.

11. Breastfeeding Network (1998) *Thrush and Breastfeeding.* London: Breastfeeding Network.

12. Breastfeeding Network (2000) *Breastfeeding and Thrush.* London: Breastfeeding Network.

13. Hale T (2000) *Medications and Mothers' Milk*, 9th edn. Amarillo: Pharmasoft.

14. Nipple vasospasm – a manifestation of Raynaud's phenomenon and a preventable cause of breastfeeding failure. http://www.gp.org.au/cls/raynaud.html (1998).

15. Royal College of Midwives (1991) Antenatal and postnatal considerations. In: *Successful Breastfeeding*, 2nd edn. London: Churchill Livingstone, pp. 53–59.

16. World Health Organization (2000) *Mastitis. Causes and Management.* WHO/FCH/CAH/00.13. Geneva: WHO.

17. Sigman M, Burke KL, Swarner OW (1989) Effects of microwaving human milk: changes in IgA content and bacterial count. *J Am Diet Assoc* **89**: 690–692.

18. Woolridge M, Baum D, Drewitt RF (1980) Effect of a traditional and of a new nipple shield on sucking patterns and milk flow. *Early Hum Dev* **4**: 357–364.

19. Auerbach KG (1990) The effect of nipple shields on maternal milk volume. *JOGNN* **19**: 419–427.

20. *Matt and Mandy: a solution for breastfeeding attachment through co-bathing* [video] (1994) Melbourne: Heather Harris.

21. Brigham M (1996) Mothers' reports of the outcome of nipple shield use. *J Hum Lact* **12**: 291–297 (see also writer's comments in *MIDIRS Midwifery Digest* (1997) **7**: 269 [abstract]).

22. Wilson-Clay B, Brigham M (1996) Clinical use of silicone nipple shields. *J Hum Lact* **12**: 279–285.

The milk supply

In most circumstances a mother has the potential to produce sufficient milk to exclusively breastfeed a term, healthy baby for the first 6 months of his life,[1] and thereafter to make a substantial contribution to her baby's nutrition for at least the next 2 years.[2] It is curious, therefore, that the most common universal reason mothers give for stopping breast-feeding early is that they do not have enough breastmilk. Quite simply, as long as milk is regularly removed from the breast, more milk will be made to take its place. The quantity of milk can be increased by feeding or expressing more often; by making sure that the milk is removed efficiently from all the lobes of the breast; and by ensuring that the baby's attachment to the breast, and the positioning used to maintain it, are good. In this way the milk supply (the milk available to the baby or which can be expressed) should be able to continue for as long as the mother wants.

The breast is a highly efficient gland – so why do some mothers have difficulty with their milk supply, particularly those whose babies require special care?

5.1 TOO LITTLE MILK

There are several causes of low milk production (milk synthesis at the cellular level) and subsequently a low milk supply. Usually a combination of factors is responsible. Only 3–4% of mothers have a genuine breastmilk insufficiency,[3] caused by a lack of functioning glandular tissue or other physiological factors.

5.1.1 Physical factors that may interfere with milk production

◆ The possibility of retained placenta should be suspected, if the milk supply is difficult to initiate in the first few days following delivery.[4] It is always worth checking the mother's notes to see if the placenta was complete at delivery. Any large blood clots passed should be reported to and examined by the maternity staff.

◆ Inverted nipples can be an indication that the mother has a reduced number of lobes in the breast, which may result in a reduced output of milk.[5] In this case it is important for the mother to be given all the information from this section. She should be encouraged to produce as much milk as she can, so that it can be used in conjunction with any formula milk the baby may also need to be given.

◆ Breast surgery, in which the lobes, the ductal system or the nerve supply have been partially removed or damaged, will affect the milk production.

◆ Low maternal levels of thyroid hormones are associated with low milk production.[6]

◆ Severe haemorrhage after delivery can damage the pituitary gland causing loss of the anterior pituitary hormones – therefore prolactin is no longer produced. This condition is known as Sheehan's syndrome.

◆ An acute illness may temporarily reduce milk production.

◆ Another pregnancy!

Any milk a mother expresses is valuable.

Stress

A mother with baby on a neonatal or paediatric unit commonly experiences a fluctuating milk supply. This appears to be related to the 'ups and downs' of her baby's medical condition. Periods of acute stress usually coincide with an apparent temporary reduction in the mother's milk supply – evidenced by her expressing less than normal or in extreme cases not being able to express anything at all. This is because her oxytocin is temporarily inhibited by her stress. The milk *is* in the breast, but the temporary inhibition of the let-down reflex, triggered by oxytocin, stops the myoepithelial cells from contracting and pushing the milk into the ducts. It is understandable why this apparent decrease or lack of milk flow can make a mother even more anxious, causing her to worry about her milk supply. Thus, a vicious circle is created very quickly. The mother requires constant reassurance and support. Once she is aware that a temporary inhibition of her let-down reflex may occur, it is easier for her to cope with this physical reaction to her baby's condition. It helps if she knows this is not a real reduction in her milk production – as long as she continues to express regularly.

Growth spurts

During the first 2–4 months after delivery, there may be times when the milk supply seems inadequate for about 24–48 hours. The baby may become irritable and want to feed more frequently, sometimes up to 14 times in 24 hours.[7] This is common, and usually coincides with the baby having a period of rapid growth.[8] If a mother understands that her baby needs her breast for extra comfort at this time, when he may be feeling uncomfortable, and also needs additional milk, she will know that as long as she lets her baby suckle more often, her body will adjust to his new requirements. The baby will settle back into a feeding pattern of around 8–10 times in 24 hours. This usually happens within 48 hours, although some babies may take up to a week to settle properly. It is not uncommon for mothers of term babies to experience this first around the 5–6 week period, which, incidentally, also coincides with one of the periods when mothers often give up breastfeeding.[9] Mothers of preterm babies may find that their babies also go through unsettled periods corresponding to growth spurts, but their occurrence is less predictable than with term babies. A mother who is aware of these periods when her baby will want to be fed more often, and knows why her baby is irritable, will also know that her milk supply is sufficient for his needs.

Mothers who have a low milk supply, for which none of the above factors is thought to be the cause, may find some of the following suggestions helpful. Mothers with a genuine problem of milk production may also benefit from these suggestions, which are aimed at optimizing their milk supply. However, they may continue to have a low milk supply, and the baby may still require supplementation with a formula milk or human banked milk.

5.1.2 Helpful suggestions

To prepare for feeding or expressing

1. Before feeding or expressing, the mother should try to sit down for 5–10 minutes (longer if possible!) with a warm drink and listen to some favourite music, preferably restful – music by Mozart is reputedly good for relaxing the mind! She may find it relaxing to massage her breasts gently.

2. Tell the mother that if her partner massages her breasts or otherwise stimulates them, this may have a positive result on encouraging milk production. This is helpful just before breastfeeding or expressing her milk.

3. Nipple stimulation is also important because it directly encourages release of prolactin and oxytocin.

4. Encourage the mother's partner or a friend to massage her back (see section 3.6).

5. Whenever possible the mother should have the opportunity to hold her baby in her arms with skin-to-skin contact. Even if he is in the intensive care unit and is ventilated, as long as he is stable he will benefit from being held close and hearing his mother's heartbeat. One of the

advantages to small babies of being held in this way is that they maintain their body temperature more efficiently with skin contact. It has the overall benefit of stimulating the mother's milk production.[10]

About feeding

1. Feed the baby on demand, even if this means more frequently than is indicated on his fluid chart (as long as he is not fluid-restricted). This will help build up the mother's milk production and supply.

2. If the mother is in a mother-and-baby room and her baby is able to breastfeed without any problem, advise her to go to bed with her baby, so that she can feed him whenever he wants. Encourage the mother to have as much skin contact as possible with her baby. She can do this whether her baby is just beginning to learn to breastfeed, or breastfeeding is already well established.

3. The breastfeeding supplementer can help build up the milk supply by encouraging the baby to suckle and stimulate the breast.

About expression

1. If the mother has previously produced good volumes of milk, reassure her that she will again.

2. Express from warm breasts in a warm room. If a mother is cold, advise her to have a warm bath or shower prior to massage and expression, or to bathe the breasts in warm water, or to put a warm towel or flannel on the breasts prior to massaging and expression.

3. If the mother is using a hand pump, suggest she changes to an electric pump or hand-expression.

4. If using an electric pump, check the mother's technique. Make sure she is expressing for long enough; that she is alternating between breasts every few minutes; and encourage her to increase expressing to every 2–3 hours for 24–48 hours, i.e. 10–12 times or more. Advise her to express at least twice in the night, with no long intervals between sessions.

5. Advise the mother to express from both breasts after a feed. This is particularly important if the baby is preterm and has a weak suck, which may not stimulate the mother's milk production efficiently.

6. An alternative to the previous point is to let the mother express her milk for 24–48 hours rather than let her baby breastfeed. After each expression, encourage the baby to suck on the emptied breast.[11] The baby can be given milk either by cup or oral gastric tube. This may also be a useful method for a preterm baby, who needs practice at the breast, but is still receiving most of his feeds by tube.

7. Warn the mother that when she is discharged from hospital she may notice a temporary reduction in her milk supply, but she should continue to express as previously. The reduction may be a result of the

mother not expressing as frequently or for as long as when she was in hospital.

8. Metoclopromide, domperidone in small doses, or oxytocin nasal spray (in some countries) are sometimes recommended to stimulate the milk supply, and are worth considering if other advice consistently fails.[12,13] These drugs have to be prescribed.

General advice

1. Advise the mother to rest as much as possible, both during the day and at night.

2. The mother may need to rethink her priorities. Housework, for example, may have to be given a secondary position for a while, and offers of help should not be refused! It may be impossible for her to have the same daily routines she had before she was pregnant.

3. Check any drugs that the mother may be taking. If she is a smoker, make sure that she smokes after feeding or expressing, not before.

4. Check whether the mother has resumed taking an oral contraceptive; if so, make certain she is on the progestogen-only pill ('mini-pill'). If she has been given the combined pill, the oestrogen content will diminish her milk supply.[14] In this case, tell the mother to contact her doctor immediately or, if necessary, you should contact her doctor to ensure she is prescribed the correct contraceptive drug. This may be one cause of a diminishing milk supply at around 6 weeks.

5. A homeopathic remedy for diminished milk supply is 'Mother tincture' (*Urtica urens*). This is obtainable from a homeopathic pharmacy. However, if a mother wishes to use homeopathic remedies it is important she consults a registered homeopath. Acupuncture may also be worth considering, in which case it is important to consult a registered acupuncturist. (The appendix contains the addresses of professional organizations which can provide further advice.)

Reassure the mother that a diminished milk supply is only a temporary problem.

5.2 TOO MUCH MILK, A FORCEFUL LET-DOWN REFLEX AND LEAKING BREASTS

Having more breastmilk than is necessary may seem to be an advantage, but it can equally be a source of concern.

5.2.1 Too much milk

◆ Some mothers with an excessive milk production will have already noticed that milk was leaking for several weeks before the birth of their baby. After delivery the milk continues to leak in generous amounts between breastfeeds or expressions. It can be acutely embarrassing, particularly when the milk leaks on to her clothes. It may take several weeks or months for the milk supply to diminish sufficiently for leaking to stop, and for some mothers it may only stop once breastfeeding ceases. Interestingly, it is seen more often in first-time mothers, and may not happen with future pregnancies.

◆ Mothers with an excessive milk production who are expressing their milk may easily obtain well over a litre and a half per day from the first week after delivery. If the mother has a preterm baby, she will be expressing considerably more than her baby needs. It is then important that she follows the regimen outlined in section 5.3.2. This will ensure her baby receives sufficient fat-rich hind-milk for his energy needs.

◆ Another option for the mother, if she fills more than one bottle at each expression, is to put the milk into a single container after the expression and thoroughly stir it, to mix it, before putting it back into separate bottles for storage. This ensures that one bottle of milk is not qualitatively different from the other.

◆ If the mother is breastfeeding her baby, she may find it necessary to express some milk before she attaches her baby, so that he receives some hind-milk as well as fore-milk.

◆ The mother can take the baby off the breast when she feels the let-down, then reattach him when the flow of milk slows. She can catch the milk in a drip catcher, a cup, or with a clean, dry cloth or breast pad.

◆ An excessive milk production usually has no pathological cause. However, if the mother is distressed by the problem she should discuss it with her doctor. There are some extremely rare medical conditions affecting prolactin which can result in excessive milk production, and these may need to be excluded.

For many mothers, milk production is **not excessive** but is greater than her baby's needs. This can be very frustrating as her baby may be gaining weight too slowly and having supplements of low-birthweight formula added to his expressed milk, even though there is plenty of the mother's milk in the freezer. Again, the mother should follow the formula in section 5.3.2 to ensure he receives adequate amounts of fat-rich hind-milk for his needs.

For the majority of mothers an abundant milk supply is not a permanent problem. If the mother's milk supply continues to be moderately abundant beyond the first or second week after birth, and she is breastfeeding a healthy, term baby (who may simply need antibiotics because his mother had premature rupture of her membranes) it may indicate poor attachment. Continual stimulation of the nipple area stimulates prolactin and more milk is produced. She should avoid wearing clothes or underwear that constantly are loose against the nipple.

Sometimes when a baby is breastfeeding for all or some of his feeds, at around 33–36 weeks' gestation or post-conception age, or he is weakened by illness, his mother may have more milk than he needs; this may continue beyond the first few days of lactation.

What can the mother do if the milk production is excessive?

1. Wear a well-fitting brassière.
2. Avoid any kind of nipple or breast stimulation.
3. Lightly wrap her baby up for a feed so that he cannot touch her breasts.
4. Check that there is nothing in her diet or any medicines that may stimulate her milk production.

Other suggestions

1. If the breastmilk tends to come too fast for the baby, a different position for feeding may be beneficial. The flow may be slowed if the mother lies on her back or reclines in a chair, with her baby positioned on her abdomen, so he can easily take the breast. The baby's head can be supported with the mother's hand on his forehead (Fig. 5.1).
2. A nipple shield may be useful, as this is known to reduce the supply of milk.
3. It takes approximately 6 weeks to completely establish breastfeeding, by which time this problem has usually resolved. It is important for a mother to know that it is unlikely to be a permanent condition.

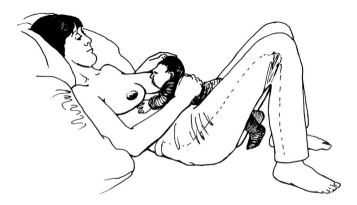

Figure 5.1 Positioning a baby when the mother has a very abundant milk flow.

4. Hand-expression reduces the amount of milk obtained, if expression of breastmilk continues to be necessary.

Mothers who have to express breastmilk for a baby in a neonatal or paediatric unit, and who choose to use a mechanical pump, may find that they are able to express volumes well in excess of their baby's needs. When expression has to be maintained for several weeks, the mother's milk production may still be very high when her baby is ready to breastfeed. Many mothers find that it takes several days for their milk production to adjust to the needs of the baby rather than to the pump (even though the mother has stopped using the pump). If this is thought to be the probable cause of an excess milk supply, the suggested ways of weaning a mother off a mechanical pump are appropriate (see section 3.4).

5.2.2 A forceful let-down reflex

Some mothers with an abundant milk supply find that the milk sprays spontaneously from the breast when feeding is about to take place. This may indicate a very active let-down reflex. The milk may fill the baby's mouth too quickly, causing him to choke and panic. He may 'fight' at the breast. If the baby is preterm, weak or just beginning to learn to breastfeed, this can make him choke and increases the risk of aspiration. To avoid this:

◆ The mother may find using a position in which she leans back in her chair, lies in a semi-reclining position or lies flat on her bed will help slow the flow.
◆ The mother can express some milk prior to feeding to slow the flow (20–30 mL is usually sufficient). In addition, by expressing some milk at the beginning of the feed, she will ensure that she is not left uncomfortably full at the end of the feed. This will also enable the baby to obtain more of the fat-rich hind-milk, which will be more satisfying than a feed high in fore-milk.

In any situation where the mother produces more milk than her baby needs, there is a risk that the baby will have a low-fat diet consisting mostly of fore-milk because he is already full before he gets to the fat-rich hind-milk. The lactose content is higher in fore-milk and can be a cause of colic. Expressing some milk before the feed as suggested above may prevent this from happening.

5.2.3 Leaking breasts

Leaking breasts can be very distressing to mothers. Leaking does not occur necessarily because there is too much milk, but because the tiny muscles in the nipple are weak. An overenthusiastic let-down reflex can cause leaking from the breasts, at or before a feed. This can occur when a mother hears her baby cry, when she sees her baby, or from some other personal trigger mechanism.

When leaking is considered to be a problem:

◆ It can be stopped by the mother applying pressure to the nipples with her arms across her chest or with the heel of her hand (Figs 5.2 and 5.3). This should be done as soon as the let-down or tingling sensation, or leaking, is felt.
◆ It may be helped by splashing cold water on the nipples or gently rubbing them with an ice-cube every 3–4 hours.
◆ Although Woolwich shells are useful, they should only be worn during a feed or expression, to collect milk draining from the other breast, as they can encourage leaking by causing pressure on the milk sinuses.
◆ If a brassière is worn it should be well-fitting to prevent stimulation of the nipple.
◆ Sometimes wearing loose, lightweight clothing helps because there is less nipple stimulation.

Breast pads can be worn to absorb leaking milk, but should be abandoned if the nipples become sore or cracked, particularly if the pads are lined with plastic.

This problem usually resolves itself within a few weeks. It is rarely a permanent condition.

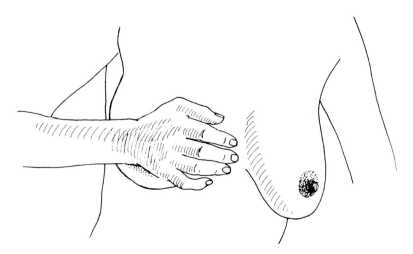

Figure 5.2 Hand position to prevent milk leakage.

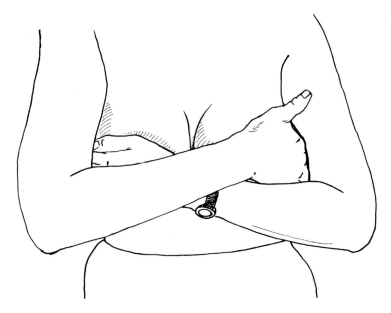

Figure 5.3 The position of the arms to prevent milk leakage.

5.3 EXPRESSION OF THE FAT-RICH HIND-MILK

The quality of the milk given to a preterm, low-birthweight or ill baby is of paramount importance to his growth and wellbeing. How a mother expresses her milk may possibly influence the quality of the breastmilk her baby receives. To optimize the collection of milk that is most beneficial to a baby, it is necessary to look at basic aspects of expression.

A baby requires a balance of the nutrients in breastmilk so that he receives adequate amounts of fore-milk and of hind-milk, with its higher fat content. A potential problem may arise, however, if the mother expresses much more milk than her baby requires – a not unusual occurrence when she uses an electric pump. This may result in the baby receiving milk which has a low hind-milk (fat) content. If as a result the baby's growth begins to slow, a low-birthweight or standard formula may be introduced to his diet. However, it is possible, if the mother has a sufficiently good milk supply, to express it in a way that ensures a balance of the fore-milk and hind-milk. Thus, the baby receives the benefit of the mother's milk without needing as much additional formula milk or fortification.[15] Making use of the fat-rich hind-milk can improve a baby's weight gain,[16] although it is necessary to check regularly on the baby's protein intake.[17]

A fat-rich hind-milk regimen can be used with babies as young as 25 weeks.[15–17] To optimise the collection of milk that is most beneficial to a baby, it is necessary to look at some basic aspects of expression.

5.3.1 Using milk rich in hind-milk to promote growth in the preterm baby

To improve the weight gain and growth of a preterm baby using the mother's own breastmilk, the following information is needed:

1. An estimate of the baby's **current** 24-hour fluid (milk) requirement.
2. A record of how much milk the mother expressed over the **last** 24-hour period.

The assumption is made that the mother will express approximately the same amount of breastmilk as in the previous 24 hours. It is important for her to keep a record of the amounts she has obtained at each expression in a 24-hour period for at least 3 days prior to this, to see how much variability there is in her supply.

If the amount of milk expressed by the mother is **more** than the baby's requirements, portioning breastmilk with a higher fat-rich hind-milk content is possible. To do this, the mother needs to have at least two bottles for each expression. These should be clearly labelled to distinguish between the bottle containing the fore-milk and that containing the fat-rich hind-milk.

5.3.2 The formula

The formula is the mother's total amount of expressed breastmilk produced in the previous 24 hours, minus the baby's current total milk requirements.

The following example shows how to obtain the fat-rich hind-milk. The amounts used in the example are only given to illustrate the method. The actual 'fraction' of the mother's milk to be expressed into bottle 1 and bottle 2 will vary with each mother/baby pair and sometimes also from day to day – insofar as the baby's fluid requirements change on a daily basis.

The method is simple and straightforward, and mothers very quickly become experts at knowing how much milk to put into each bottle, as long as you tell them how much milk the baby needs at each feed.

Example

Information to be collected

1. The amounts the mother expressed at each of seven expressions are recorded on a chart designed for the purpose. The 24-hour total was 425 mL. (These figures are examples only.)

The sums

2. The mother produced a total of 425 mL of breastmilk in the **previous** 24-hour period.
3. Her baby requires 200 mL of milk in the **coming** 24 hours.
4. The requirement of 200 mL is approximately half of 425 mL.

The daily expression schedule

5. At each of the mother's seven expressions during the **coming** 24 hours the mother needs to express approximately half of her milk, from both breasts, into the bottles labelled '1'. These will contain milk with a higher level of fore-milk.
6. The actual amount she expresses into bottle 1 each time is based on the amount she expressed at that time on the previous day. In her case she will halve the amount.
7. She can indicate in marker pen on the side of the bottles to show the amount that should be expressed into bottle 1.
8. The remainder of the milk from both breasts will be expressed into the bottles labelled '2'. These bottles will contain both fore-milk and hind-milk. There is likely to be more milk in these bottles than in the bottles labelled '1'.
9. The milk in the bottles labelled '2' will be given to the baby. The milk in the bottles labelled '1' will all be frozen.

The daily sums

Baby's current requirements = 200 mL per 24 hours.
Mother's previous 24-hour total = 425 mL.
   At each expression on the previous day, the mother expressed the following amounts:

1. Early morning   80 mL
2. Mid-morning   75 mL
3. Lunchtime   68 mL
4. Mid-afternoon   60 mL
5. Early evening   50 mL
6. Bedtime   50 mL
7. During the night   42 mL

The total amounts of milk to go into the '1' bottles, from both breasts, are:

1. 40 mL
2. 35 mL
3. 35 mL
4. 30 mL
5. 25 mL
6. 25 mL
7. 20 mL

All the remaining milk at each expression should be expressed into the bottles labelled '2'. This milk is given to the baby.

Important points to remember when expressing for fat-rich hind-milk

◆ Bottle 1 should have milk in it from *both* breasts, and so should bottle 2.
◆ The total amounts expressed into bottle 1 and bottle 2 will vary with each expression, although the proportions will be constant throughout the day. In the example given the proportion was approximately half of the milk in each bottle (see example); but it could have been one-third and two-thirds if the baby had required 400 mL and the mother expressed a total of 600 mL.
◆ The bottles should be clearly labelled. Coloured labels are useful, not only are they easily seen and identifiable, but they are also easy for mothers to use. For example, a blue label could be attached to bottle 1, and a yellow label to bottle 2. The bottles with the yellow labels containing the richer milk are given to the baby.
◆ Ask the mother to keep a record of the amounts of milk she is expressing into bottle 1 and bottle 2. A chart designed for the purpose is very easy to make.
◆ Record on the baby's weight chart when feeding with the fat-rich hind-milk was commenced. Check on the baby's progress. If you have any worries about his growth or weight gain, please discuss it with the doctors.
◆ Write out the regimen for the mother, so that she knows exactly what she must do and approximately how much she should express.

Important! It is necessary to check the record of the mother's expression totals daily. If the 24-hour total begins to diminish to a point where a surplus is no longer possible, **stop** expressing in this way and commence expressing the full amount into one bottle only, until there is an excess of milk again. Give the expressed milk the mother produces as normal.

5.3.3 Promotion of weight gain in a baby who is breastfeeding

If a mother has an adequate milk supply but the weight gain of her baby is poor or static, or the baby is preterm or compromised by a clinical condition, expression of some fore-milk **before** a feed begins will ensure the baby is able to obtain milk containing the hind-milk during a breastfeed. The baby can then be offered the expressed fore-milk by cup if he is still thirsty. The amount of milk that should be expressed is as follows:

1. On day 1, express 10–20 mL of fore-milk from each breast into a bottle or a cup, before each breastfeed.
2. Then breastfeed normally.
3. Give the expressed milk by cup, if the baby requires more after a breastfeed.
4. On days 2–5, express less milk prior to each breastfeed.
5. If after this regimen the weight gain begins to slow again, repeat steps 1–4.

As the baby matures he will take more milk from the mother and she will not need to express before each feed.

5.4 THE NORMAL GROWTH OF THE BREASTFED BABY

A number of studies have shown that the growth patterns of breastfed and formula-fed babies are different.[18–21] In the first 2–3 months after birth, breastfed babies put on weight more rapidly than formula-fed babies, but from the third or fourth months, they tend to grow more slowly.[22–24] In the mid-1990s a new set of charts was produced for measuring the growth of children from 20 weeks' gestation through to young adults of 20 years.[25] Interestingly, because feeding practices have changed over the last 2 decades, and more babies needing neonatal and paediatric care now receive breastmilk, the data used to construct the charts for preterm babies reflect more accurately the growth of breastfed babies than was previously the case. For the charts of babies from 40 weeks' gestation the amount of breastfeeding data is less, but the new charts are also closer to a breastfed pattern than previous ones.

Since 1994 the World Health Organization, together with a number of other United Nations agencies and national institutions, has been involved in a multinational study to develop growth reference data to reflect the growth patterns of healthy, breastfed babies and young children.[26] These data will be considered to show the 'normal' growth of babies against which other feeding methods will be measured. Importantly, this will lead to the development of growth charts that *will* accurately reflect the growth of breastfed babies, from birth to 24 months.

5.5 WEIGHT LOSS AND TEST WEIGHING

5.5.1 Initial weight loss and future weight gain

A certain amount of weight loss is considered **normal** in the first few days of life. A term, healthy baby can lose up to 10% of his birthweight within the first 3–5 days, regaining it by 8–12 days after delivery. This is so common that now many healthy babies may be weighed at birth and then not weighed again until they are 7 or 8 days old, unless there is any cause for concern.

The majority of babies requiring special care, however, need to be monitored far more regularly. Many of these babies will lose larger amounts of weight in the initial period after birth. This is because, in addition to the 'normal' weight loss, which is mostly connected to adjustments in the baby's total body water at birth, their initial weight loss is exacerbated by extra energy requirements needed to fight infection or illness, maintaining their body temperature, and other metabolic requirements. A baby with a low-birthweight, but who is the correct length for his gestational age (these babies usually look rather skinny!) may lose little weight at birth. These babies are often very hungry and may want to be fed more frequently than babies whose initial birthweight is appropriate for their gestational age.

In contrast, the initial weight loss of a preterm baby may be extreme. This is related to his gestational age and weight at birth; the lower these are, the greater the initial weight loss is likely to be. How quickly he regains his birthweight will depend upon how low his gestational age is, his condition, and his original birthweight.[27] Some babies requiring special care may take up to 3 weeks before they really begin to gain weight.

It is interesting that some term, healthy babies born at home have been observed to have no initial weight loss,[28] possibly as a result of the environment they were born into: a warm room, avoiding any initial heat loss, immediate and sustained skin-to-skin contact and access to the breast. These mothers were relaxed during labour and afterwards. It may be that larger volumes of colostrum are produced when a mother is relaxed. Colostrum has a higher osmotic pressure than mature milk, minimizing the water loss which accounts for much of the initial weight loss at birth.[29,30]

If a term, healthy breastfeeding baby loses 10% or more of his birthweight, it may be necessary to investigate why, and look particularly closely at his attachment and positioning.

Once birthweight is regained, a normal term baby should double his birthweight by the fifth to sixth month. After this the baby gains approximately 80–100 g per week and should have trebled his birthweight by the end of his first year. This pattern of rapid weight gain in the first few months followed by a period of slower weight gain is considered the normal pattern for term, healthy babies, and is clearly seen when they breastfeed.

5.5.2 Other causes of weight loss

Weight loss may be due to:

◆ insufficient milk supply (rare)
◆ the use of expressed breastmilk with a high fore-milk content
◆ a sleepy baby, not taking sufficient milk or not waking to feed on demand
◆ incorrect positioning and attachment at the breast
◆ a preterm or ill baby lacking the energy to feed long enough to obtain sufficient breastmilk or the hind-milk
◆ timing and scheduled feeds.

5.5.3 Test weighing

Test weighing is rarely necessary and may seriously undermine the mother's confidence. The results may totally misrepresent what the baby has taken in a breastfeed, for the following reasons:

◆ The scales may not be accurate.
◆ The baby will almost certainly take different amounts at different feeds.
◆ There is no indication as to the nutritional value of the feed – a baby may have had 40 mL of fore-milk and hind-milk and be completely satisfied, or 50 mL of fore-milk and be totally unsettled: which weight would be accurate? More importantly, which baby will have had the most benefit from his feed?

If test weighing is considered necessary, it should be carried out over a 24-hour period. If it is the mother who wants the test weighing to be carried out, it is better to teach her how to recognize when her baby has had sufficient milk. If she still wishes her baby to be test weighed, the points above should be explained to her. If it is the health professionals who want the baby to be test weighed, then the question 'why?' needs to be asked, to see if there is an alternative way to obtain the information required. Is it simply a lack of confidence in the mother's milk supply or her ability to meet her baby's requirements, or is it that health professionals feel more comfortable when they can count the number of millilitres the baby has taken, and know its 'nutritional' quality.

5.6 BREAST SURGERY AND FEEDING

Breast surgery does not mean that successful breastfeeding is impossible, except where bilateral mastectomy has been performed, or where the nipples have been removed or are absent.

Successful breastfeeding is possible when:

◆ one breast has been removed but the other breast functions perfectly normally
◆ the mother's nipples have been re-sited, but the nerves and ductal system have been left intact and can function in the different position
◆ breast reduction or silicone implant surgery has been performed, as long as the nerve supply of the nipple and the ductal system necessary for lactation have been left intact (and the silicone implant is not leaking)
◆ removal of breast lumps or drainage of a breast abscess has been performed.

It is necessary to read the mother's medical notes or to contact her general practitioner to discover exactly what treatment or surgery she has previously received, particularly in the case of major breast surgery.

In situations where surgery has reduced the milk supply temporarily, the breastfeeding supplementer is invaluable until the normal functioning of the breast returns. The mother may require advice and help with relactation. Following surgery where the normal functioning of the breast is no longer possible, providing the nipples are present, 'breastfeeding' can also be achieved using the breastfeeding supplementer. A mother will need much support and encouragement (as indeed will any mother who has undergone breast surgery, for whatever reason). The establishment of a satisfactory 'breastfeeding' technique using the breastfeeding supplementer can be psychologically beneficial to the mother and the relationship she has with her baby.

5.7 RELACTATION

Having a baby on a neonatal or paediatric unit makes a mother particularly vulnerable to a variable milk supply. There are times when a baby cannot breastfeed because he is ill, or having surgery, maybe the mother is ill and a long gap has occurred during which her milk supply has stopped, or she may have started breastfeeding but her baby was unable to suckle effectively. It may be that the mother initially chose to give her baby formula milk by bottle and now wants to breastfeed, or that she is adopting a baby or is having a baby through surrogacy, but has never been pregnant. In all these cases a milk supply needs to be stimulated so that the woman can either continue or begin to breastfeed. The processes involved are:

◆ **Relactation** – the ability of a woman who has stopped breastfeeding, no matter how long ago, to start again. This is possible even if a mother has not breastfed for many months or even years.[31]
◆ **Induced lactation** – the ability of a woman who has never been pregnant to produce breastmilk and breastfeed.[32,33]

For relactation or induced lactation to work the woman needs to have a strong desire to feed her baby, she has to be well motivated, and needs considerable support for her efforts. Many people find the idea of relactation and induced lactation strange. Relactation, however, is common in many parts of the world, and where it is accepted as a normal physiological occurrence it happens far more easily.

For mothers of babies who require special care, relactation is more commonly the need than is induced lactation. In both cases the methods of stimulating milk production are almost the same.

5.7.1 Stimulation of relactation

The stimulation required for a woman to produce breastmilk is of two kinds: mechanical and hormonal.

Mechanical stimulation

Methods of mechanical stimulation include:

◆ the suckling of a baby (the best stimulation of all)
◆ breast and nipple massage
◆ pump or hand-expression; a pump may be more effective than hand-expression (dual pumping is worth trying)
◆ a 'borrowed' baby – from a friend or relative
◆ a partner to stimulate the breasts.

Hormonal stimulation

◆ Prolactin is produced when the woman's nipples are stimulated.
◆ In a non-lactating breast, prolactin stimulates growth of the alveoli (see section 1.3).
◆ Oxytocin really only works once milk is secreted into the breast. However, the psychological state of the woman is so important to oxytocin working properly that she needs to be well supported from the beginning.

Holding the baby with plenty of skin-to-skin contact will encourage mechanical and hormonal stimulation of the breast.

5.7.2 What to do to relactate or induce lactation

If the baby is willing to suck

◆ Breastfeed as often as possible, every 1–2 hours, at least 8–12 times in 24 hours.
◆ Sleep with the baby.
◆ Encourage the baby to suck as long as possible. Use both breasts, at least 10–15 minutes on each side at each breastfeed.
◆ Ensure good attachment and positioning. Leaning and lying positions may be helpful.
◆ Check on the baby's intake. Check on urine output by weighing the nappies. Weigh each nappy dry first; each one may have a slightly different weight.
◆ Relactation may occur earlier when lactation has only recently stopped.
◆ Do not use bottles, pacifiers or nipple shields.
◆ If supplements are necessary, use a cup, gastric tube or breastfeeding supplementer.

Continue the above regimen until milk can be hand-expressed, and the baby is growing adequately without supplementation. Milk may begin to appear between 1 week and 6 weeks after the stimulation and/or drug treatment begins.[34] An adequate milk supply may take several weeks to achieve.

Women may additionally require metoclopramide, 10 mg three times a day, for at least 7 days.[35] Some women may also find additional breast stimulation from an electric pump is necessary.

If the baby is unwilling to suck

◆ Ensure the baby is not ill.
◆ Increase the amount of skin-to-skin contact. Encourage the woman to carry her baby in a sling next to her breast (this is how 'kangaroo care' works).
◆ Offer the breast regularly.
◆ Use a breastfeeding supplementer to encourage the baby to breastfeed.
◆ Stimulate the breast and nipple – by hand or by pump.
◆ Do not use bottles, pacifiers or nipple shields. However, if the baby has been using a dummy or has had a bottle feed, lightly rub a dummy or bottle teat over the nipple and areola. The baby may respond to the smell.

◆ Encourage the mother and baby to have a bath together. They will need to be supervised. The water should be comfortably warm, without being too hot. It should reach the mother's lower chest when she leans back against the bath. She should have her baby placed on her chest between her breasts so that he can easily reach the nipples and areola to feed. The carer with the mother and baby should gently pour water over the baby's back so that he remains warm. This may help the baby to 'rediscover' the breast.

If a baby is unable to go to the breast

1. A mother who has no baby to put to the breast may find she has sufficient stimulation from hand-expression or from an electric pump to encourage the milk supply to build up, particularly if she has had a good milk supply in the past few weeks. Dual pumping may be particularly beneficial to her.
2. She should express every 2 hours until she is able to express adequate volumes of milk for her baby's requirements, or until she is happy with the amounts expressed.
3. Treatment with metoclopramide should be considered.

Induced lactation

The mother needs to know that most women can produce sufficient volumes of milk to partially satisfy their baby's needs within 6 weeks of commencing treatment and pump stimulation. However, she may never produce all the milk her baby requires. The milk produced is considered to be equivalent to mature breastmilk.[36,37]

Composition of milk in relactation and induced lactation

◆ There is no significant difference in the milk of a mother who relactates or induces lactation compared with the mature breastmilk of a mother who has experienced no difficulties.
◆ It has been observed that women who have never been pregnant produce no colostrums.[36] However, at 5 days their milk had similar amounts of total protein, alpha-lactalbumin and immunoglobulin A.

5.7.3 Drug treatments

Some women, especially those who have never been pregnant, or who have not breastfed for a very long time (weeks or months), may find that milk does not appear despite following the above measures. They may find the following drugs are useful. The woman should always consult her doctor, as these are all prescription drugs. The main drug treatments use metoclopramide or chlorpromazine, which increase prolactin release.

Metoclopramide

◆ Dose: 10 mg three times a day for 7–14 days.
◆ Unless a mother is well supported after the drug treatment finishes, her milk supply may noticeably decrease.

Chlorpromazine

◆ Dose: 25–100 mg three times a day for 7 days.
◆ In most cases milk is produced 5–10 days after commencement.

Other drugs

Other drugs that appear to help some mothers include:

◆ domperidone[38]
◆ sulpiride
◆ oxytocin nasal spray.

Drugs should only be used for relactation if no milk has appeared after 2 weeks of trying the methods outlined above. All these drugs have some side-effects (see the *British National Formulary* or the book by Tom Hale, *Medication and Mothers' Milk*; more information is given in the appendix).

Hormones

◆ Oestrogens, progesterone or hormonal contraceptives may be used to induce lactation in women who have never been pregnant. These drugs act in a similar way to the hormones of pregnancy, by stimulating the development and growth of the alveoli.
◆ Breastmilk usually begins a few days after the hormones stop and the baby is able to suckle at the breast.

5.8 THE MOTHER'S DIET AND FLUIDS

Mothers tend to feel hungrier and thirstier during lactation, and they will benefit if they eat when they feel hungry and drink when they feel thirsty.

Many mothers with babies on a neonatal or paediatric unit miss meals altogether, have no appetite, or only have snacks when there is time and when they remember. While it is quite understandable that this should happen, a mother needs to take care of herself, and may need gentle encouragement and persuasion to eat and drink regularly. Even though physiologically there may be no evidence to link diet with milk volume, a combination of stress, missed meals and a different routine appears to have the effect of temporarily reducing the mother's milk supply, possibly because she is not expressing as often as she needs to, or for as long at each session, thereby draining her breasts less effectively. If a mother is not given sufficient support at this time, her milk production may be permanently affected as her confidence becomes undermined.

A balanced, healthy diet is ideal. It is essential, when giving advice to mothers, to find out what their normal diet and eating and drinking habits are, and to offer advice around this information, if necessary. A diet designed for weight loss is generally inappropriate for a lactating mother. Regular eating habits should be maintained with breakfast, a nutritious lunch and an evening meal. Some mothers also find that they need a snack mid-morning, mid-afternoon and mid-evening. Some mothers prefer smaller, more frequent meals during the day and evening; this is quite satisfactory and may have the advantage of ensuring an even energy intake.

Many babies become more restless and are perceived to be more demanding towards the evening. This may be because the mother's milk production is naturally lessened towards the end of the day. (Mothers who express milk will usually obtain more milk in the morning and less as the day proceeds.) Sometimes it helps a mother if she has a snack in the late afternoon and mid-evening. Small snacks of high energy value can be beneficial in providing the body with sustainable energy to produce milk; foods such as halva, nutritional supplements ('build-ups'), dried fruits and cheese appear to be useful. In addition, it will greatly benefit the mother if she can have practical help with any tasks that have to be done in the evenings, for example, cooking and coping with other children after school or at bedtimes.

There is no evidence to suggest that any foods should be avoided altogether, but some mothers may observe that certain foods appear to affect their baby's digestion (this may happen with foods that have a short growing season and may be eaten in some quantity, e.g. strawberries).

A mother should drink plenty (but not excessively) so that she is not thirsty. Do not recommend an amount by the litre or jug, or the mother may become very uncomfortable, particularly in the first few days following delivery. She should have a drink beside her when breastfeeding, as this is when she is likely to be thirsty. Milk does not have to be taken to produce milk, but it is a good source of protein and energy. It is probably best for a mother to avoid drinking many cups of strong coffee. Caffeine is a drug and may cause a preterm baby to appear restless.

REFERENCES

1. World Health Organization (2001) The optimal duration of exclusive breastfeeding. Results of a WHO systematic review. Press release 7, 2 April 2001.

2. World Health Organization (1993) *Breast-feeding. The Technical Basis and Recommendations for Action.* Saadeh RJ, Labbock MH, Cooney KA, Koniz-Booher P (eds). WHO/NUT/MCH/93.1. Geneva: WHO.
3. Neifert MR (1983) Infant problems in breastfeeding. In: *Lactation.* Neville MC, Neifert MC (eds). New York: Plenum Press.
4. World Health Organization (1989) Infant feeding: the physiological basis. *WHO Bull* **67**(suppl.): 21.
5. Lawrence RA (1987) The management of lactation as a physiological process. *Clin Perinatol Breastfeeding* **14**: 1–10.
6. Riordan J, Auerbach KG (1993) Maternal health. In: *Breastfeeding and Human Lactation.* Riordan J, Auerbach KG (eds). London: Jones & Bartlett, p. 355.
7. Powers NG (1999) Slow weight gain and low milk supply in the breastfeeding dyad. In: *Clinics in Perinatology. Clinical Aspects of Human Milk and Lactation.* Wagner CL, Purohit DM (eds). London: WB Saunders, pp. 399–430.
8. Countryman BA (1991) Self-care. In: *A Practical Guide to Breastfeeding.* Riordan J (ed.). Boston: Jones & Bartlett, p. 67.
9. Office of Population Censuses and Surveys (1992) *Infant Feeding 1990.* White A, Freeth S, O'Brien M (eds). London: HMSO.
10. Hurst NM, Valentine CJ, Renfro L et al (1997) Skin-to-skin holding in the neonatal intensive care unit influences maternal milk volume. *J Perinatol* **17**: 213–217.
11. Narayan I, Mehta R, Choudhury DK et al (1991) Sucking on the 'emptied breast': non-nutritive sucking with a difference. *Arch Dis Child* **66**: 241–244.
12. Budd SC, Erdman SH, Long DM et al (1993) Improved lactation with metoclopramide. *Clin Pediatr* **32**: 53.
13. Ehrenkranz RA, Ackerman BA (1986) Metoclopramide effect on faltering milk production by mothers of premature infants. *Pediatrics* **78**: 614.
14. Tankeyoon M, Dusitsin N, Chalapati S et al (1984) Effects of hormonal contraception on milk volume and infant growth. *Contraception* **30**: 505–522.
15. Kirsten D, Bradford L (1999) Hindmilk feedings. *Neonatal Network* **18**: 68–70.
16. Lang S (1995) *Feeding and Growth Pattern of Infants in a Neonatal Unit* [data collected 1989–1990 on growth of very low-birthweight babies fed their own mother's breastmilk containing the fat-rich hind-milk fraction]. MPhil Thesis, University of Exeter.
17. Valentine CJ, Hurst NM, Schanler RJ (1994) Hindmilk improves weight gain in low-birth-weight infants fed human milk. *J Pediatr Gastroenterol Nutr* **18**: 474–477.
18. Whitehead RG, Paul AA (1984) Growth charts and the assessment of infant feeding practices in the western world and in developing countries. *Early Hum Dev* **9**: 187–207.
19. Duncan B, Schaefer C, Sibley B (1984) Reduced growth velocity in exclusively breast-fed infants. *Am J Dis Child* **138**: 309–313.
20. Dewey KG, Heinig MJ, Nommsen LA (1992) Growth of breast-fed and formula-fed infants from 0 to 18 months: the DARLING study. *Pediatrics* **92**: 1035–1041.
21. Chandra RK (1982) Physical growth of exclusively breastfed infants. *Nutr Res* **2**: 275.

22. Hitchcock NE, Coy JF (1989) The growth of healthy Australian infants in relation to infant feeding and social group. *Med J Aust* **150**: 306–311.
23. Whitehead RG, Paul AA, Cole TJ (1989) Diet and growth of healthy infants. *J Hum Nutr Diet* **2**: 73–84.
24. Butte NF, Garza C, Smith EO (1984) Human milk intake and growth in exclusively breast-fed infants. *J Paediatr* **104**: 187–195.
25. Child Growth Foundation. *Boys/Girls Growth Charts.* United Kingdom cross-sectional reference data: 1996/1.
26. World Health Organization (2000) *Nutrition for Health and Development. A Global Agenda for Combating Malnutrition.* WHO/NHD/00.6. Geneva: WHO, pp. 62–63.
27. Muhudhia SO, Musoke R (1989) Postnatal weight gain of exclusively breastfed preterm African infants. *J Trop Paediatr* **35**: 241–244.
28. Odent M (1990) The unknown human infant. *J Hum Lact* **6**: 6–8.
29. World Health Organization (1989) Infant feeding: the physiological basis. *WHO Bull* **67**(suppl.): 9–15.
30. Bustemante SA, Jacobs P, Gaines JA (1983) Body weight, static and dynamic skinfold thickness in small premature infants during the first month of life. *Early Hum Dev* **8**: 217–224.
31. World Health Organization (1998) *Relactation. A Review of Experience and Recommendations for Practice.* WHO/CHS/CAH/98.14. Geneva: WHO.
32. Hormann E (1977) Breastfeeding the adopted baby. *Birth Fam J* **4**: 165.
33. Philips V (1971) Establishment of lactation for the breastfeeding of an adopted baby. *Res Bull Nurs Mothers Assoc Austr* 4.
34. Lawrence R (1994) Induced lactation and relactation (including nursing the adopted baby) and cross nursing. In: *Breastfeeding: A Guide to the Medical Profession,* 4th edn. London: Mosby, pp. 555–574.
35. Lewis PJ, Devenish C, Kahn C (1980) Controlled trial of metoclopramide in the initiation of breastfeeding. *Br J Clin Pharmacol* **9**: 217.
36. Kleinman R, Jacobson L, Hormann E et al (1980) Protein values of milk samples from mothers without biological pregnancies. *J Pediatr* **67**: 612.
37. Kulski JK, Hartmann PE, Saint WJ et al (1981) Changes in the milk composition of non-puerperal women. *Am J Obstet Gynecol* **139**: 597.
38. Da Silva OP, Knoppert DC, Angelini MM et al (2001) Effect of domperidone on milk production in mothers of premature newborns: a randomised, double blind, placebo controlled trial. *CMAJ* **164**: 17–21.

Breastfeeding the vulnerable baby

6.1 TONGUE-TIE (ANKYLOGLOSSIA)

Tongue-tie can sometimes interfere with a term baby's ability to breast-feed. In extreme cases the baby's tongue is not rounded at the tip; instead, when an attempt is made to protrude it, the tip is M-shaped and does not come out further than the lips. In preterm babies, a degree of apparent tongue-tie is not uncommon. As the baby grows, the problem usually corrects itself. However, there is a very small percentage of term babies with tongue-tie who cannot touch their hard palate with the tip of their tongue or protrude their tongue over their bottom lip. These are the babies who may require minor surgery to release the tie.

If you suspect the septum (frenulum) beneath the baby's tongue is restricting its movement, tell the doctors. Make sure a breastfeed has been carefully observed to see exactly how the baby uses his tongue.

If a mother has sore nipples yet the attachment appears to be good, check inside the baby's mouth to see if he has tongue-tie, and look to see how far he can extend his tongue. Some babies do not have any problems attaching to the breast and breastfeeding well. It is helpful if the mother's areola and nipple are soft at the time of attachment, so that they can be drawn far enough into the mouth for the tongue not to damage the nipple. The mother may find positions in which her breast falls into her baby's mouth helpful. Tell the mother to make sure her baby extends his tongue as far as possible before attachment.

6.2 CLEFT LIP AND PALATE

There is no doubt that breastfeeding presents a challenge to the mother of a baby with either a cleft lip, a cleft palate, or both. It requires patience, perseverance and a great deal of commitment from the parents and from the medical and nursing staff, indeed from everyone involved in the care of the mother and baby.

It is very important to support this mother if she decides to breast-feed. The mother–baby relationship may be enhanced, the baby will receive the benefits of the breastmilk, and both mother and baby may derive a great deal of comfort from the skin contact breastfeeding inevitably requires.

One of the potential long-term benefits of breastfeeding for the baby is the positive effect on the development of the palatal muscles, which are enhanced through the mechanical action of breastfeeding itself. This helps to maintain the patency of the eustachian tubes, thereby reducing the likelihood of serious ear problems. These babies have an increased risk of otitis media and continuing ear problems as they grow older.[1]

6.2.1 Cleft lip

As long as the cleft is only in the baby's lip, breastfeeding should be possible.

6.2.2 Cleft palate

Even a small cleft in the palate may cause considerable problems. If the baby cannot maintain a vacuum between his tongue and the palate, he cannot make a teat out of the breast, which is a prerequisite for breast-feeding.

Where the cleft is in the baby's hard palate, breastfeeding presents an additional challenge and will certainly require more patience. The area between the hard and soft palate is important in the stimulation of the sucking reflex. This may be diminished in a baby with a lesion in this part of the palate. It helps if the mother's nipple and areola are soft and pliable enough to go easily into the baby's mouth, and the mother has an efficient let-down reflex. It is, therefore, crucial for the mother to be instructed on how to avoid breast engorgement.

The positioning and attachment of the baby are vital to successful breastfeeding. Different breastfeeding positions should be tried, for it is unlikely that any one conventional position will be appropriate for all of these babies. Suggested alternative positions may include:

◆ The baby in a sitting position, supported across his mother's lap, or supported along side his mother's side with his legs pointing towards the mother's back, as in the underarm position (Figs 6.1 and 6.2).
◆ The baby on his back with the mother leaning over to let the breast fall directly into his mouth. This position is useful for a term baby who has a mature swallow reflex (Fig. 6.3).
◆ Leaning and lying positions will also be useful, as they ensure the maximum amount of breast tissue can fall as far as possible into the baby's mouth.

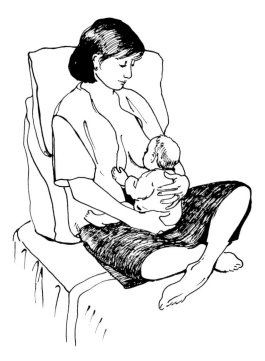

Figure 6.1 A position for feeding a baby with a cleft abnormality.

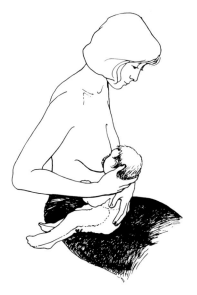

Figure 6.2 A position for feeding a baby with a cleft abnormality.

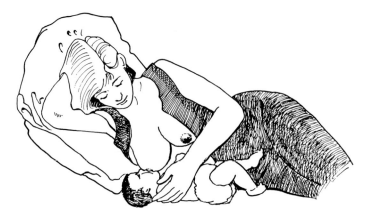

Figure 6.3 A position for feeding a baby with a cleft abnormality.

6.2.3 Cleft lip and palate

With a unilateral cleft lip and palate, breastfeeding may be possible. It will require imagination and flexibility in technique. All possible feeding positions should be tried, including those described above, until a suitable one is found. To enhance attachment at the breast and create a seal around the baby's mouth, the mother may find it helpful, once the breast tissue is far enough in the baby's mouth, to:

◆ put the edge of her hand or her index finger just under her breast
◆ gently push the breast tissue upwards so that it fills the baby's cleft
◆ maintain this pressure on the breast tissue until the feed ends.

If the baby has a cleft lip only, this will help him as well. The mother should be encouraged to express regularly to keep her breasts as soft as possible.

It may take several days for the mother and the baby to establish an acceptable breastfeeding technique, and even then it is highly probable that she will have to supplement her baby with an additional feeding method, until surgical closure of the lip and palate takes place.

6.2.4 The establishment of breastfeeding

It may help a mother who wishes to breastfeed, if the initial few weeks following birth can be devoted to the establishment of breastfeeding – without bottles being introduced.

◆ Once the mother has the baby positioned at the breast, even if she is still experimenting with positions, she should gently hand-express a little milk into his mouth. This often results in the baby wanting more, whether he is preterm or term.

◆ The baby should be allowed to experiment with suckling at the breast as often as possible. It is not uncommon in these early days for a baby to appear frustrated at the breast. One important cause may be that the nipple, or the teat of a bottle, may have gone through the cleft into the nasopharyngeal space, causing him difficulty in breathing and swallowing – and to panic, which is alarming for the mother. It may take time to overcome this problem, for to suck effectively the baby has to compress the nipple or teat between two firm surfaces. The nipple or teat may need to be angled in the baby's mouth to achieve this. Breastfeeding may for this reason be an easier option for a baby, as the mother's let-down reflex will allow milk to flow with the minimum of compression. It is important for the mother to express after feeding, to ensure the breasts receive adequate stimulation. Alternatively, the mother may find that expressing a small quantity of milk **before** feeding may ensure the baby obtains the fat-rich hind-milk, thus helping with weight gain.

The mother must accept that during this time she may have to supplement her baby's feeding with an alternative method. This needs to be introduced while the mother is in hospital, partly to assess its suitability, and partly to give the parents time to practise. Bottles do not have to be used; a cup, cup and spoon, or the breastfeeding supplementer may be used instead.[2,3] Gastric tubes should be removed as soon as possible, as they may hinder a baby's ability to swallow efficiently. Term babies should not require gastric tubes unless there are other problems present at birth.

Even if breastfeeding is established in an acceptable way to the mother and her baby, an additional method of feeding may still be necessary until corrective surgery has taken place. Breastfeeding alone may not be able to supply the baby with sufficient volumes of milk to ensure his growth is adequate. This is because the baby is unable to drain the milk sinuses efficiently. It is important, therefore, to monitor his growth carefully in the first few days and weeks after breastfeeding is established. Weights should be recorded every 2 days or so. If they are satisfactory, then there is no need to supplement the baby with additional fluids. However, if the weight remains static or weight loss occurs on more than two consecutive occasions, then an additional feeding method will need to be considered. Do not test weigh this baby after each feed; it will invariably undermine the mother's confidence.

It is important to support this mother. It is possible for her to succeed, but she will need help. Therefore, any way of maintaining the mother's milk supply, continuing with the breastfeeding so far established, and using an acceptable additional feeding method should be encouraged. Time at the breast may be an important positive experience for the baby, particularly if the mother is to establish total breastfeeding once surgery has been performed.

A baby with a bilateral cleft lip and/or palate may also be able to feed from the breast, although this is uncommon. Those who are not able to suckle can still be fed expressed breastmilk by cup,[2–4] or by cup and spoon. The baby can also taste and lick any milk expressed onto the nipple, or take milk directly expressed into his mouth from the breast.

6.2.5 If breastfeeding is not established

If breastfeeding has not been established, or looks unlikely to become so, at the end of a reasonable period of time (for example, 3 weeks), bottle-feeding may be introduced. This does not mean the mother should not persevere with breastfeeding as well. Expressed breastmilk can be given by bottle; a variety of teats may need to be experimented with, such as a Habermann teat, a cannon teat, a 'lamb's teat' (which is long and soft) or an ordinary teat.

6.2.6 Support groups

The date of any future corrective surgery may also have an influence on the mother's ability to maintain her commitment to breastfeeding and continued expression of breastmilk. If surgery is likely within the first 6 months of life, a baby may well be able to breastfeed afterwards, with the perseverance and patience of the mother. There are several cases where this has occurred, and the mother should contact one of the breastfeeding support groups (addresses in the appendix). All have counsellors who will be able to provide the mother with the help and support she will definitely require, and may have specialist counsellors who have experience of this situation. The Cleft Lip and Palate Association (CLAPA) is the specific support group for parents of babies with a cleft lip and/or palate, and is able to give additional help and advice with feeding (the address is also in the appendix). There is also a beautifully produced booklet called *Give Us A Little Time*, by Christa Herzog-Isler and Dr Klaus Honigmann (see appendix).

6.2.7 General advice

- Make sure this mother knows how to hand-express. Teach her how to avoid engorgement.
- Feed the baby in a semi-upright or sitting position, or in any position that allows him to satisfactorily complete a feed. The mother lying down with her baby alongside may be a useful position, as the breast

can, with gravity, fall far enough into her baby's mouth for the milk to be swallowed, without going into his nose.

◆ Make sure the baby can suck well, by giving him plenty of practice of sucking on a knuckle or fist, or a clean finger, rather than on a dummy. This is important so that he becomes used to sucking on an object that is not static in the mouth.

◆ Encourage the baby to open his mouth widely. The mother can make use of his rooting reflex by gently teasing his cheek or bottom lip with the nipple.

◆ Always express a small amount of milk on to the nipple prior to attaching the baby at the breast. Direct expression will help him to respond to the taste of breastmilk initially, and may help the milk to flow more easily.

◆ Introduce any additional feeding method as early as possible, so the parents have plenty of practice of using it. The cup, cup and spoon, and the breastfeeding supplementer should all be considered for use.

◆ Breastfeeding may be more successful if a baby's initial hunger is met with his mother's preferred alternative feeding method, and then he is attached to the breast.

◆ The baby may need 'winding' more frequently than other babies.

◆ This mother and baby should be discharged when her milk supply is established, the baby's position and attachment at the breast are satisfactory, and the alternative method of feeding being used presents no danger to him.

◆ Ensure the parents are aware of the importance of monitoring their baby's weight and growth regularly.

6.3 BELL'S PALSY AND BREASTFEEDING

If part of a baby's face is temporarily or permanently paralysed, this can cause problems in the commencement and establishment of successful breastfeeding or bottle-feeding.

Bell's palsy is caused by pressure on the seventh cranial nerve. It can arise in three main ways:

◆ Most commonly, from delivery by forceps: this causes temporary facial paralysis, which usually begins to improve within 24–48 hours, but can last for up to 6 weeks.

◆ Pressure in utero on the nerve from the pelvic bones: this may cause permanent damage depending upon how long the pressure has existed.

◆ Abnormal nerve development causing permanent facial palsy.

The seventh cranial nerve affects movement in the face and the anterior portion of the tongue, possibly interfering with taste. However, the nerves supplying facial sensation and therefore the rooting reflex, movement of the tongue, palate and generally the nerves involved in sucking and breathing are not affected. The main problems are:

◆ an inability to form a seal with the mouth around the areola or teat
◆ an inability to open the mouth as widely as necessary in breastfeeding.

To overcome these problems:

1. Express a little milk onto the nipple at the start of the feed.
2. Position the baby so that the paralysed part of his face is facing away from the breast, therefore ensuring maximum stimulation for opening the mouth widely.
3. Hold the baby in the underarm position so that the mother has maximum control of his head. Alternatively, the mother may find having her baby lying beside her, so that the breast falls directly into his mouth, a useful position.
4. With the mother's free hand, she can gently hold the baby's chin down to encourage him to open his mouth just wide enough to ensure correct attachment. Make sure his tongue is extended out of his mouth before attachment is attempted. (Pulling the chin too far down will cause the tongue to be drawn into the back of the baby's mouth – try it yourself!)

The mother can initially express milk directly into her baby's mouth; this may encourage him to respond to the smell and taste of the milk. If the problem is temporary, always let the baby try to breastfeed first of all. If this is unsuccessful, the mother should express her milk and give it to him by cup.

A cup may be very useful if the palsy is permanent, although it will also be important to encourage the development of the sucking reflex. A Habermann teat may be useful in this situation.

6.4 BREASTFEEDING THE BABY WITH BREATHING AND HEART PROBLEMS

To successfully breastfeed, the suck, swallow and breathing reflexes have to be well coordinated. A number of factors can interfere with the efficiency of these reflexes. In any baby with breathing or heart problems an assessment should be made prior to feeding. This should include:

◆ respiratory rate
◆ heart rate

- signs of breathing difficulty
- colour
- transcutaneous oxygen level.

During a feed the following assessment should be made:

- length of sucking bursts
- the baby's ability to remain attached to the breast
- the baby's position at the breast
- respiratory and heart rate
- colour
- transcutaneous oxygen level.

A high respiratory rate, for example, can impede the coordination of the suck, swallow and breathing reflexes. Therefore any baby exhibiting nasal flaring, chest wall retraction or grunting should not be breastfed until his condition is more stable and his respirations less laboured. A baby with stridor or noisy breathing may have difficulty breathing in between sucking because of a narrowed airway. This may be because there is a problem with the shape of the airway, or simply a blocked nose, or there is a nasogastric tube in place. It is important to check whether there is a simple solution to this problem or whether oral feeding is possible, so that tube feeds are not given unnecessarily.

In a normal pattern of suckling the suck–swallow sequence is repeated approximately once a second. The baby continuously sucks and swallows in bursts of approximately 10–30 sucks with pauses in between. During these suck–swallow bursts the baby also breathes, usually following the swallow. The pauses vary in length but in a term, healthy baby are usually quite brief. It is thought that during these pauses the baby is able to recover from any respiratory compromise resulting from swallowing. Therefore a baby with heart or breathing problems or who is ill may have longer pauses between bursts. Breastfeeding has the advantage that for most babies, when suckling stops, the milk also stops flowing.

The length of the suck–swallow bursts may indicate how well the baby is coping with the feeding process. Short bursts following attachment, with no initial quick sucking sequence at the beginning of the feed to start the let-down reflex, may indicate that the baby is unable to cope with suppressing breathing during frequent swallowing. Long bursts without any breathing in between are likely to result in a reduced oxygen level and may also cause a slow heart rate. In both cases the cause may be immaturity or lack of energy and the resultant lack of organisation needed to ensure the suck–swallow reflexes are well coordinated. As a baby's condition improves or he matures this coordination improves along with his breastfeeding.

Evidence suggests that breastfeeding is less stressful to preterm babies than bottle-feeding, and that temperature and oxygen levels also remain more stable throughout breastfeeding.[5-7] This is partly because a baby who breastfeeds can pace his own feeding, in time and quantity, whereas with bottle-feeding, it is the person giving the feed who may influence the pace, in a number of direct ways (e.g. gently shaking the bottle when the baby stops sucking, or making the hole in the teat bigger). A breast-fed baby is held close to his mother's breast, with its familiar scents, taste and sounds. All of these factors are an advantage for a baby compromised by respiratory or heart problems, and who needs to conserve his energy.

A baby dependent on oxygen given via a nasal cannula can usually breastfeed without too many difficulties. His head should be supported so that it is extended enough for his nose not to be pressed into the breast tissue. This ensures the little tubes in his nose are not uncomfortably positioned. The underarm position may be the most appropriate to achieve this (Fig. 6.4).

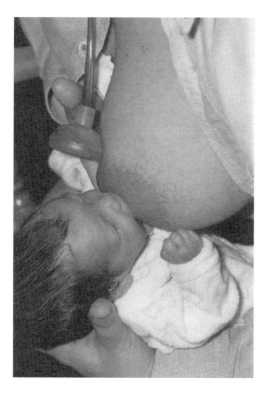

Figure 6.4 The position and breast attachment of a baby requiring oxygen therapy (photograph courtesy of the North Staffs Neonatal Unit).

If a baby is receiving ambient oxygen in his incubator, he rarely has a problem, when out with his mother, as long as oxygen is given via a funnel placed over her shoulder, near the baby's nose.

If a baby requires more than 50% oxygen in a headbox, it is better to wait until the oxygen requirement comes down to 30–35% before attempting to breastfeed. An oxygen requirement of 30–35% will not harm an otherwise healthy baby being held by his mother for a short time with oxygen delivered via a funnel. He can usually cope with having a little milk expressed directly into his mouth, or an attempt at breastfeeding. It may be necessary to keep this baby attached to an oxygen saturation monitor during his time out of the incubator.

A baby who is tachypnoeic and agitated as well is best left to rest. However, if he has no other symptoms apart from tachypnoea he may benefit from being held close to his mother and allowed to breastfeed if he wishes. The decision to do this must depend upon the baby's clinical condition and the agreement of the doctors.

6.5 MULTIPLE BIRTHS

Mothers are well able to produce sufficient milk for twins or triplets, without supplementation being necessary. If a mother has more than three babies at one time she may wish to use a formula milk as well, or consider contacting a milk bank to see if it is possible to use human milk for supplementation (UK Milk Bank Association address and telephone number are given in the appendix). Documented cases of mothers feeding quadruplets indicate that milk supply is often not the problem.[8] Milk supply is much more likely to be maintained if the mother is well supported and has assistance with other domestic needs.

6.6 THE PRETERM BABY

Until a preterm baby gives some indication that he is ready to take milk directly from the breast, the mother must express milk so that she can maintain her milk production and supply.

In addition to touching and talking to her baby, the expressing of milk is the most important thing that a mother who wishes to breastfeed can do (particularly for the preterm or ill baby). It is milk unique to that baby and cannot be provided by anyone other than the mother. It is important for her to be aware of this. It is also worth asking mothers 'particularly of babies born between 24 weeks and 32 weeks' who wish to bottle-feed, if they will consider expressing their breastmilk until the baby can tolerate gastric bolus feeds of a formula milk and oral feeds from a bottle.

Whenever possible, the mother should be encouraged to hold her baby. Skin-to-skin contact is ideal.[9] This gives the baby the opportunity to familiarize himself with the mother's scent and the feel of the breast, and encourages bonding in difficult circumstances. It also helps stimulate the mother's milk supply and gives unlimited access to the breast. A preterm baby of around 32 weeks who is stable can be supported inside the mother's clothing (in a sling) and 'worn' while the mother is on the neonatal unit. The baby can sleep and be fed next to the mother's skin. This is how 'kangaroo care' works. Its benefits are a calm baby and a mother who lactates more easily.

Between 32 weeks and 34 weeks and sometimes as early as 30 weeks, the baby will show signs of being more awake, of wanting to suck on anything close by, e.g. his fist, and of not being satisfied by either continuous tube feeds or intermittent feeds via the gastric tube. When this occurs, it is worth encouraging the mother to express directly into the baby's mouth, and for cup feeds to be gradually introduced. To give the baby the experience of non-nutritive sucking, encourage him to suck on the breast **after** the mother has expressed, or during tube feeds.

It is important that the mother is prepared for the sequence of events that her preterm (or ill) baby is likely to go through in order to establish breastfeeding, so that she does not expect too much in the early stages. She should also know how she can avoid problems developing during this period.

The main features of a preterm or ill baby are:

◆ a weak suck
◆ the baby may tire easily
◆ a lack of coordination in sucking, swallowing and breathing
◆ a degree of immaturity or regression in behaviour.

6.6.1 Overcoming the problems

All these problems can be overcome by some or all of the following:

◆ At each opportunity when the mother is in the unit, she should, depending upon her baby's condition, be able to hold him. If milk is hand-expressed onto the nipple, the baby should be able to taste it. If he wants to try suckling, make sure positioning and attachment are correct so that he has no difficulty in taking her milk.

◆ The mother or her helper can gently massage the breast towards the nipple, encouraging the milk flow. Never try to force the baby to suckle. Suckling will eventually occur, but only when he is ready – patience and perseverance are the secret!

◆ Correct positioning and attachment of the baby are vital to successful breastfeeding, particularly in these early stages. The mother needs to feel competent at positioning so that she can be independent of hospital staff as soon as possible. The underarm position is very useful for a small baby, where his mouth is small in relation to the nipple. In this position the mother has control of the baby's head, and can direct the nipple and areola into his mouth more easily. The baby can be encouraged to open his mouth widely by gentle brushing of his cheek or lips with the mother's nipple, or by slight pressure on his chin to open his mouth. Too much pressure will be counterproductive as it will cause the tongue to be drawn too far back into his mouth.

The mother may find another position more suitable for her. As long as she can feed successfully, and can maintain the position, she should use the position she is most comfortable using.

❖ A preterm (or ill) baby will initially tire easily. It is useful if the mother starts the milk flow by hand-expression before attaching him to the breast. The baby will organize his sucking pattern differently to a more mature baby. Initially, sucking is for short periods with frequent rests in between. These rests may be quite long. Gradually, sucking will last for longer periods before resting occurs. If the baby is attached to the breast, encourage his mother to keep him in position and not to move him just because there is a long pause between suckling or because he appears to be asleep. These very long pauses are completely normal at this stage. If the baby is asleep, gently change his position, if he does not stir sufficiently for the feed to continue, then it is best to finish the session and let him rest. If, however, he is still awake but lacks the energy to finish his feed at the breast, he can be given a cup feed.

❖ Frequent attempts to make a preterm baby breastfeed will be counterproductive. It is better to have one concerted effort during the day when the conditions are right, i.e. the baby is awake, hungry and wanting to suckle. At other times, the mother should be encouraged to hold the baby close while he is being tube-fed – but allowing the baby to take milk from the breast in his own time. The baby's readiness to breastfeed becomes obvious from the response shown to his mother, as time continues. Gradually, the mother should be encouraged to be present at more feed times. Before discharge she should be able to stay in the unit for one or two nights if possible, or until she is confident that her baby can feed well. This period is also useful to help wean the mother off the pump, if she has been expressing for a long period.

❖ For many preterm babies, when they are initially learning to breastfeed, supplementation or replacement of feeds is necessary via a nasal or oral gastric tube or a cup, with either expressed breastmilk or a formula milk. Low-birthweight formulae are sometimes prescribed by the doctors when the baby's weight gain is very slow or static. However, if the mother has an abundant milk supply, suggest she follows the 'hind-milk' regimen. The baby should then begin to gain weight more quickly. If the mother hand-expresses her milk, do not divide the milk into separate bottles. Use it all, making certain the bottle is shaken to distribute the fat content evenly before using any milk. If any formula milk is used, mix it with the mother's own milk, because absorption is likely to be more efficient.

◆ Gastric tubes should be removed as quickly as possible, as they may delay the coordination of the suck and swallow reflex.[10] Cup-feeding is useful because it allows the baby to take what he wants and pace himself. It is also a useful method of supplementing a baby after a breastfeed if this is necessary. It gives the baby the taste of the milk and the added stimulation that this provides, such as exercise of the tongue and jaw muscles, and release of lingual lipases to aid fat digestion. Cup-feeding can be safely used before the baby is able to breastfeed. Parents should be shown how to use this method of feeding.

◆ If a baby is taking milk at the breast, providing that it is more than just a few sucks, wait till the baby indicates that he is hungry before supplementing or breastfeeding again. In the initial few feeds, it may be necessary to give a baby a supplementary feed after the breastfeed. In this case, it is better to wait half an hour to an hour before giving the tube feed. Small babies often require 2-hourly feeds and, if there are no contraindications, it is better to wait until the next feed is due before any supplementation is given. This depends on the circumstances of each individual baby. The mother should express milk from both of her breasts, until the baby is able to drain the breasts efficiently himself.

◆ Once a baby is taking two-thirds of his feeds via the breast, he may appear to go for longer or shorter periods than the schedule laid down by a unit on a feed chart. This is normal behaviour for a baby. A preterm baby may well require more frequent feeds until his stomach grows. Gradually he will develop his own routine. It is useful for a baby to receive regular (i.e. 3-hourly) tube feeds overnight so that his mother has more flexibility during the daytime.

Weighing the baby every second day is a useful way of assessing his progress, once he is able to regulate his own intake and feed times.

6.7 THE VENTILATED BABY

A baby who is being ventilated will be able to receive his mother's expressed breastmilk via a gastric tube. The mother's milk can also be used for her baby's mouth care (rather than using sterile water). This will be pleasant for him and may additionally stimulate some lingual lipase activity.

A term or preterm ventilated baby who is stable can be held by his mother (or his father) with skin-to-skin contact. This can help to relax the mother and, encourages her milk flow.[11] It is also valuable for either of the parents to be able to touch and comfort their baby, when he is still so fragile and so in need of their special touch and closeness.

6.8 THE JAUNDICED BABY

6.8.1 Physiological or idiopathic jaundice

Jaundice is a common condition in babies who are preterm, infected or bruised, following a difficult delivery – particularly after a forceps delivery or after a vacuum extraction. Jaundice is also more common among babies who are breastfed compared with those who are formula-fed,[12,13] although this may reflect problems with breastfeeding practice.

The bilirubin level in physiological jaundice usually reaches its peak 3–4 days after delivery.

6.8.2 How to reduce the development of jaundice in the first few days after birth

1. Breastfeeding or the administration of expressed breastmilk (if necessary) should be commenced as soon after birth as possible.
2. Colostrum should be given to a baby because it aids the quick passage of meconium, due to its laxative effect. It thus prevents the high level of bilirubin contained in meconium being reabsorbed and further increasing the level of jaundice.[14]
3. Demand feeding and good positioning and attachment of the baby at the breast, from birth, ensure that he receives sufficient colostrum and milk, to prevent or lessen the development of jaundice.

The following two points are important for term babies with a bilirubin level just below the level requiring phototherapy:

◆ The baby should be nursed beside his mother, either in the postnatal ward or in the neonatal unit.
◆ The baby should be fed whenever he wants to be.

6.8.3 Pathological or haemolytic jaundice

Pathological jaundice may occur as a result of haemolysis of the baby's blood, owing to an ABO blood incompatability. It may also result from drug therapy given to the baby and – on rare occasions – from some maternal disease states.

The jaundice level peaks at around 24 hours after birth, but jaundice may be present from soon after delivery in both term and preterm babies. In serious cases the baby will require an exchange transfusion. Phototherapy will also be necessary. Breastmilk should be given to meet his fluid needs and breastfeeding should continue when the baby is sufficiently awake to feed.

6.8.4 Phototherapy and feeding method

◆ When phototherapy is prescribed, additional fluids may be necessary to prevent dehydration. However, for a term or preterm baby who wakes and demands his feed, and breastfeeds well, supplementary fluids will not be required.

◆ More frequent feeds may be demanded by the jaundiced baby to counteract any diarrhoea or increased thirst; therefore, any time schedule should be flexible enough to allow true demand feeding – even if this means feeding every 1–2 hours.

◆ Nasal or oral gastric tubes should not be passed unless the baby is very sleepy. Cup-feeding may be a better method of supplementing a baby because a mother can give the cup feed and hold her baby closely as well. This may stimulate him to wake-up.

◆ If a baby is very sleepy when jaundiced, 3-hourly feeds may be necessary, even though he may not be able to breastfeed efficiently. The breast should be offered first of all; if he does not appear interested or is too sleepy, a cup can be offered. If this is also unsuccessful, the feed should be given by a gastric tube, which is then removed after the feed (so that it does not interfere with his potential suckling ability at the next feed).

◆ If a breastfeed is successful, supplementary feeding is not necessary. It can be helpful to the baby if his mother expresses some milk onto her nipple before he begins his feed.

◆ A jaundiced baby who is receiving phototherapy and is not waking for feeds or is feeding inadequately may require additional fluids via a gastric tube. If he will take a cup, this should be offered. Babies of 36 weeks or less may be more susceptible to being sleepy before feeds. Milk should be given as the supplementary or replacement fluid, not water or dextrose. The protein in the milk lines the baby's gut, decreasing the reabsorption of unconjugated bilirubin. This does not happen with water or dextrose, and increased levels of bilirubin may result.

◆ If a mother is unable to express sufficient breastmilk, a formula milk should be used together with her expressed milk, as the two will work more effectively together than formula milk alone.

◆ The breastfeeding supplementer may help the baby to feed more effectively.

6.8.5 Breastmilk jaundice

The cause of breastmilk jaundice is poorly understood. However, it is the most likely explanation of prolonged jaundice in the newborn breastfed baby (that is, jaundice that continues beyond the first week). It is thought that the baby reacts to an unknown substance in the mother's milk. This substance causes some enzyme activity in the baby's liver, which results in a slower breakdown and secretion of bilirubin.

The bilirubin level peaks at around 5–8 days after birth and high levels may persist for several weeks (sometimes as long as 16 weeks), during which time the baby remains jaundiced. It is not necessary to stop breastfeeding, and there are no recorded cases of kernicterus with breastmilk jaundice. Occasionally, on medical advice, breastfeeding may be stopped for 12–24 hours (a fall in the serum bilirubin level during this period usually confirms the diagnosis). In this case, the mother should express her milk and freeze it until she is able to resume normal breastfeeding. The baby's serum bilirubin concentration is likely to rise again when breastfeeding is resumed, but generally not to the levels previously reached.[15]

6.9 THE UNSETTLED BABY

There are numerous reasons for a baby being unsettled at the breast or after a feed. Many of these causes, although not connected to breast-feeding, can have a negative effect on its success. They include:

◆ the mother's emotional state (tense or anxious)
◆ the baby may have a dirty nappy or a sore bottom
◆ the baby may be too cold or too hot
◆ the baby may have wind or colic
◆ the baby may feel insecure and require swaddling
◆ the baby may simply want to be cuddled or entertained
◆ the baby may have thrush and, therefore, have a sore mouth
◆ too many people may have handled the baby (for example he may have been held by too many visitors), causing him to be overstimulated
◆ the baby may be in a smoky atmosphere, if either parent or someone nearby is smoking.

Reasons connected to breastfeeding may include:

◆ poor positioning and attachment at the breast
◆ the baby's nose may be blocked by nasal secretions
◆ the baby may be squashed against the breast, causing him to panic if he cannot breathe easily

- the let-down reflex may be very strong, causing the milk to flow too quickly
- the mother of a preterm baby may have more milk than the baby requires, causing him to take mostly fore-milk so that, though full, he still feels hungry; colic may develop as a result
- insufficient milk
- the mother may have eaten something that has affected the taste of her milk (interestingly, it appears that the mother's diet, and the effect it has on the smell and taste of her milk, may influence her baby's readiness to accept certain complementary foods)[16]
- The mother's menstrual periods may have begun, which can similarly affect the taste of her milk.

Note: make sure that the baby does not suffer from tongue-tie. This will certainly interfere with breastfeeding and cause the baby to be agitated. Some simple solutions may include:

1. Playing calming music while feeding.
2. Breastfeeding in a warm room with soft lighting.
3. Checking the baby's position and attachment are correct at the breast.
4. The baby may be soothed by a warm bath.
5. Stroking or massaging the baby with baby oil. This will calm both mother and baby.
6. Using a 'shell' or 'white noise' tape. These are commercial tapes or devices (the shell) which play a continual sound supposed to resemble the womb sounds. They are put close to the baby and are reported to calm him. (Vacuum cleaners and car engines are supposed to have a similar effect on a baby!) If these tapes are used, they appear to be most effective if played to the baby from birth.
7. A small tape recorder can be put into the incubator or cot. A tape of the mother's and/or father's voice can be played, or a tape of music that was played while the mother was pregnant.
8. Place a used breast pad in the incubator or cot near the baby, so that he can be comforted by the familiar smell.
9. Eliminate any obvious dietary reason for the breastmilk being less palatable to the baby.

6.9.1 To help re-establish breastfeeding

For some babies the reason they refuse to breastfeed is far from obvious, and then another approach may be called for. In such cases, under-standing how a baby responds to the breast at the time of birth can help to restore his desire to breastfeed. This is also true if it is necessary to break any patterns of behaviour that may have caused breast refusal, such as pressure on the head from someone helping the mother with attachment and positioning.

◆ Encourage skin contact. Allow the baby to explore the breast in his own time.
◆ Give the baby either a complete feed or half a feed of expressed breastmilk by cup, before the skin contact begins. This ensures the skin contact is unhurried, without the pressure to feed.
◆ Give the baby 10–15 mL of milk by cup prior to feeding, to calm him.
◆ Encourage the mother and baby to bath together.[17]
◆ Avoid the use of nipple shields, dummies, bottles and teats, and finger feeding. All of these can interfere with a preterm or ill baby learning the skills he needs for breastfeeding.

Do not time feeds!

6.10 BLOOD GLUCOSE AND THE BREASTFED BABY

Many babies requiring special care are at particular risk of developing low blood glucose levels. Our aim should be to prevent these levels from becoming abnormally low and the baby developing 'clinical' hypoglycaemia, with its attendant risks of neurological damage, which remain a concern with vulnerable babies.[18] The importance of breastfeeding or expressed breastmilk in helping to maintain stable and adequate blood glucose levels should not be underestimated – neither should the skills and patience required to help mothers at a particularly difficult time.

The relationship between the normal physiological adaptations, which take place at birth and breastfeeding in the term, healthy newborn, help to put into context the difficulties that babies requiring special care may experience.

6.10.1 The 'metabolic adaptation' of the term, healthy newborn baby

◆ At birth a baby has to make a sudden transition from being continuously nourished by his mother, via the placenta, to having intermittent milk feeds and using his own body stores for energy.
◆ After birth the baby's blood glucose level naturally falls, and is at its lowest in the first 1–2 hours after delivery.
◆ During the first 2–3 days blood glucose levels remain low, until breastfeeding is established.

◆ In response to these lower glucose levels at birth, the baby generates ketones from fat stores built up in the last trimester of pregnancy. Ketones provide an **alternative fuel to glucose**.

◆ Importantly, ketones protect the baby's brain from any potential harm from having a low blood glucose level.[19]

◆ The process of generating and using alternative fuels is called **metabolic adaptation**.

Postnatal care of the healthy, term newborn baby

After delivery, the baby should be dried thoroughly and held next to his mother's breast with skin-to-skin contact. This keeps him warm and encourages him to breastfeed. Thereafter, the baby should feed whenever he is hungry. It is common in the first days of life for a baby to have no set feeding pattern; he may sleep for long periods and feed only a few times. This should not cause any problems for a baby who is well, as long as his temperature, colour, breathing pattern and muscle tone are all normal and he is not dehydrated – and when he is breastfeeding, he is well attached and positioned. He will require no other fluids; colostrum will meet his needs until his mother's milk supply increases. Therefore, according to Hawdon et al, healthy, full-term infants do not require blood glucose monitoring, as normal metabolic adaptation ensures provision of alternative fuels.[20,21]

It should be remembered that hypoglycaemia is a characteristic of neonatal illness or a baby's failure to adapt to extrauterine life, it is not a medical condition in itself. Therefore, a healthy, term baby should not become clinically hypoglycaemic from apparent 'underfeeding',[19] unless there is a long delay in beginning feeds.

6.10.2 Which babies are at risk of hypoglycaemia?

Breastfeeding and the mother's expressed breastmilk are so important to the initial wellbeing of any baby, that it really cannot be emphasized enough how vital it is to support the mother to feed her baby as early as possible after delivery – or, if that is not possible, then to express colostrum so that it can be given as soon as practicable. This is especially important for the following groups of babies who are at particular risk of becoming hypoglycaemic. These babies will require careful monitoring, which should include taking accurate blood glucose measurements.

◆ Preterm and small for gestational age (SGA) babies both have reduced body stores of fat, and are at risk of a failed metabolic adaptation, resulting in low glucose and ketone levels.

◆ Babies may be under stress, because of:
  – cold (hypothermia)

– asphyxia at or before birth
– infection
– a heart condition.

These babies have difficulty generating alternative fuels.

◆ Transient high insulin levels (hyperinsulinism) are more commonly seen in babies of mothers with poorly controlled diabetes,[22] and occasionally in babies who are large for their gestational age (LGA). These babies have raised insulin levels which cause a reduction in the blood levels of glucose and ketone bodies.
◆ Inborn errors of metabolism or endocrine disorders may cause persistent hypoglycaemia. Babies suffering from these conditions may have a number of problems which interfere with metabolic adaptation.

After birth, any baby who exhibits abnormal clinical signs, such as becoming unusually drowsy, jittery, floppy, 'dusky' or whose skin looks 'blue', or any baby who suddenly becomes ill or who is feeding poorly after feeding well for a period of time, should have urgent blood glucose measurements taken and be carefully monitored.

6.10.3 What is a safe glucose level?

Hypoglycaemia is at its simplest a low level of blood glucose, which occurs when the body uses more glucose than it produces. However, there is no one single figure that defines hypoglycaemia for all groups of babies.[20] The baby's maturity and clinical condition will influence the level that is considered clinically significant. An eminent group of paediatricians have suggested the use of 'operational thresholds'.[20,23] This involves two levels: the **operational threshold**, which is defined as 'the concentration of plasma or whole blood glucose at which clinicians should consider intervention to increase the glucose level', and the **therapeutic goal**, which is 'the level of glucose that the intervention should aim to achieve' when caring for a vulnerable baby.[20] Their recommendations are outlined below.

Healthy, full-term infants

◆ Do not require blood glucose monitoring: normal metabolic adaptation ensures provision of alternative fuels.[20]

Infants with abnormal clinical signs

◆ Operational threshold – 2.5 mmol/L.
◆ Therapeutic goal – amelioration of clinical signs.

Infants at risk of disordered metabolic adaptation
- Operational threshold – persistently <2.0 mmol/L, or <1.4 mmol/L at any time.
- Therapeutic goal – 2.5 mmol/L for most, 3.3 mmol/L if hyperinsulinism suspected.[24]

6.10.4 Breastfeeding and the 'at risk' baby

This section is adapted from *Hypoglycaemia of the Newborn*, published by the World Health Organization.[19]

1. Any healthy 'at risk' baby who is able to breastfeed within the first hour of birth should have the opportunity of doing so. This should include healthy, preterm babies from around 32 weeks' gestation. The warmth of skin contact and breastfeeding will help the baby to conserve his energy levels.

2. An 'at risk' healthy newborn baby should have the opportunity of breastfeeding whenever he is hungry. However, he should not be allowed to go for longer than 3 hours between feeds.

3. If an 'at risk' baby is able to breastfeed he should have a blood glucose measurement taken around 4–6 hours after birth, before the **second** feed. If the result is below 2.6 mmol/L, supplementation with expressed breastmilk or formula milk should be considered. A further blood glucose measurement should be taken 1 hour after the feed. If the result remains below 2.6 mmol/L, intravenous glucose may be necessary.

4. If the baby cannot breastfeed at this time, he should be given any colostrum his mother can express, together with any artificial formula or donor breast milk considered necessary. This can be given by cup or gastric tube. This should start within 3 hours of birth and continue 3-hourly.

5. If a baby is unable to breastfeed because he is too immature, or his initial condition needs to be stabilized, particularly with respect to his blood glucose levels, he may require supplementary fluids in addition to the colostrum his mother has expressed. The recommended volumes of milk per day for this baby are 60 mL/kg on the first day, 90 mL/kg on the second day, 120 mL/kg on the third day and 150 mL/kg on the fourth day. If a baby can tolerate larger volumes these should be given, starting with 100 mL/kg on the first day.

6. Supplementary feeds should be either expressed breastmilk or formula milk, as these provide the baby with energy and contain fat. Breastmilk is preferred because it is thought to promote a ketogenic response and is more efficiently absorbed than formula. However, both are preferred to dextrose water, which is very low in energy.

6.11 BABIES WHO VOMIT

After a feed, a baby may spit some of the milk out of his mouth or he may dribble if he has had too much milk. It often looks a lot but in reality may only be about 5–10 mL. Most babies will do this at some time during the first few weeks after birth. Vomiting is more forceful, though may be just as innocent. Spitting and the occasional vomit will cause no loss of weight, dehydration or low urine output. Vomit, which is projectile in character, may indicate a problem exists, particularly if it persists. Two common causes of vomiting are discussed below.

6.11.1 Gastro-oesophageal reflux

Gastro-oesophageal reflux can be a worrying problem for parents. The baby persistently vomits small amounts of milk shortly after feeding, usually from the time of birth. The mother may feel there is something wrong with her milk to make her baby behave in this way. She needs to be reassured that this is a condition her baby will grow out of. The baby rarely appears to be in pain or discomfort when he vomits, though parents may notice that he has a lot of wind. Parents worry about the quantity of milk the baby vomits, but these babies usually have no weight loss. Gastro-oesophageal reflux appears to be more common in babies who have been tube-fed or previously intubated.[25] The condition gradually diminishes, though it may take several months. The parents need a great deal of support. A robust washing machine is useful!

Helpful suggestions

◆ Breastfeed the baby in an upright position, to reduce the amount of vomiting and prevent the risk of aspiration. Use the positions suggested in Fig. 6.1 or 6.2.
◆ Put the baby in a 'bouncy chair' after and between feeds to help keep him in a semi-upright position.[26]
◆ Carrying him in a sling may be useful.
◆ Give him small, frequent feeds.

6.11.2 Pyloric stenosis

Pyloric sternosis usually occurs between the second and sixth week after birth, though it can also occur earlier. Initially there is no pattern to the vomiting, but very soon it happens after each feed. The vomit is projectile in nature. Initially the baby appears to want to go back on the breast soon after; however he soon begins to lose weight and may show signs of being dehydrated. A simple surgical procedure is usually required, after which breastfeeding is usually possible as soon as the baby is comfortable (around 6–8 hours after surgery).

6.12 BOWELS AND THE BREASTFED BABY

Colostrum has a mild but nevertheless important laxative effect, which encourages the passage of meconium.[11] If it is given early and regularly to a baby, it will help prevent the development of jaundice, by preventing reabsorption of bilirubin from the meconium.

6.12.1 Colour and consistency

Meconium is the very dark, brown, black or green, thick and tarry stool, which is passed from birth. After 2–3 days, a 'changing' stool should be passed, which is brown in colour. This indicates that the baby is getting his mother's milk. This stool may be quite loose. Thereafter, the stool should be mustard-yellow in colour, soft to loose in consistency, with a slightly curdled appearance. Any change in consistency or colour is likely to indicate a change in the mother's diet.

6.12.2 Warning signs

- ◆ A term baby passing meconium at 4–5 days is clearly not getting enough milk.
- ◆ A changing stool at 4–5 days similarly may indicate a need to examine the feeding technique (such as positioning and attachment, any restriction on frequency of feeds, and the length of time the baby spends at the breast).
- ◆ A green stool may indicate that the baby is getting insufficient milk.

6.12.3 Frequency of bowel actions

Breastfed babies have little waste to excrete; therefore, they do not necessarily have a regular bowel pattern. Some babies may only pass two or three stools in a week. As long as the baby is otherwise healthy, gaining weight satisfactorily and is passing urine, there is no need to worry.

6.13 BREASTFEEDING AND HIV

There are few situations concerning breastfeeding that are as controversial as the issue of human immunodeficiency virus (HIV). The knowledge that HIV can be transmitted to a baby through his mother's milk has meant that mothers and their partners are faced with difficult choices when considering how their baby should be fed. This is hard enough when the baby is term and otherwise well, but when the baby is preterm or ill and is admitted to a neonatal unit, the situation becomes even more complex. The healthcare professionals who have to help and counsel this mother must be able to support her through a very difficult period indeed.

Many mothers who are HIV-infected quite simply choose not to breastfeed. The question then is, what practical alternatives does the mother have?

6.13.1 The mother's alternative feeding options in a neonatal unit

The options are:

◆ to give donor breastmilk obtained from a milk bank
◆ expression and pasteurization of her own milk
◆ to give formula milk.

How real are the first two options?

In areas where milk banks exist, donor breastmilk is available for babies in neonatal units.

In areas where access to donor milk is difficult, it is possible for a mother to express her own milk and for that milk to be safely pasteurized to be given to her own baby.[27] It is known that by heating breastmilk to a temperature of 57–62 °C for 30 minutes, HIV is inactivated,[28,29] along with other harmful organisms. Legitimate concerns have been raised about pasteurization and the reduction of immune components, enzymes and certain vitamins in the milk. For example, vitamin C content may be reduced by approximately one-third, lactoferrin by up to two-thirds, while 70–100% of immunoglobulin A will still be active. However, a baby in a neonatal unit is monitored closely, and his milk can be supplemented with minerals and vitamins or 'depending upon local policy' a fortifier can be added. It is also the case that not all the unique qualities of the mother's milk are destroyed even though some may be reduced – by contrast, formula milk contains almost none of these properties. Pasteurizing the mother's own milk is no different to using donor milk from a milk bank, except that the mother who is producing it may have more reason than most mothers to feel emotionally fulfilled by being able to use her own milk safely for her own baby. In some cases it may well be that milk banks are willing to undertake the pasteurization for the mother; however, a preliminary trial is in progress to look at the feasibility of individual pasteurization systems, which can be used by mothers themselves to heat-treat their own milk.[28]

Other options with potential for the future include the freeze-drying of breastmilk, so that it is available in powder form. This technology is already available in Sweden, though not necessarily for mothers with HIV infection.

6.13.2 The role of breastfeeding in the transmission of HIV

It is known that mother-to-child transmission (MTCT) of HIV can occur during pregnancy, during delivery and during breastfeeding. It appears that a baby who is preterm or low-birthweight is particularly susceptible to infection during delivery (though elective caesarean section may help to reduce this risk).[30] In addition, because the gut of a preterm or ill baby is more permeable than that of a healthy baby at term, the risk of transmission may be increased if this baby is breastfed or given his mother's raw breastmilk.

There is also concern that transmission is potentially higher where the mother has nipple and breast damage. Therefore, even if the mother chooses to express her milk, she should keep her breasts healthy and avoid as far as possible any inflammatory breast conditions.[31]

6.13.3 Can a mother with HIV ever breastfeed?

At present there is really very little information about the risk of HIV transmission through breastfeeding to preterm, small-for-dates and ill babies. Until more information becomes available, maybe we should be content with using the mother's pasteurized breastmilk, if that is what she wants. Nevertheless, it is a sad fact that there will always be some babies who will eventually test HIV positive, regardless of what precautions are taken to minimize the risks. This may be confirmed at around 2–3 months of age. In such cases, perhaps the mother should be able to hold her baby next to her breast – bearing in mind that unless she has been expressing up to this point she may not produce any milk, but both she and her baby may benefit from the mutual comfort of skin-to-skin contact.

6.13.4 The future?

There is no doubt that, as time passes, more research into breastfeeding and HIV will help us to refine the advice we can give to a mother, to help her make an informed choice about how to feed her baby. One study suggests that exclusive breastfeeding may be beneficial, rather than mixed feeding – that is, babies receive other foods or fluids in the first few months of life.[32] It may be that mixed feeding damages the baby's gut, thus increasing the amount of virus that can enter his circulation. Other research indicates that early cessation of breastfeeding at 3 months may be beneficial; and evidence is increasing that antiviral drugs given to the mother in late pregnancy or at the time of delivery, and also given to her baby in the early postnatal period, may lower the transmission rate of HIV.

Infection with HIV is a cruel diagnosis and decisions need to be made which may be difficult for a mother and a father to cope with. Breastfeeding is promoted for the vulnerable and fragile babies in our neonatal and paediatric units; but with our current knowledge, we simply have to face the fact that a baby may be safer by not feeding directly from his mother's breast – we then have an obligation to ensure that the mother and father know that breastfeeding is only one part of the nurturing process, and encourage them to show their love in the multitude of other ways we know babies respond to.

REFERENCES

1. Paradise J, Elster B, Tan L (1994) Evidence in infants with cleft palate that breast milk protects against otitis media. *Pediatrics* **94**: 853–860.
2. Lang S, Lawrence CJ, L'E Orme R (1994) Cup feeding: an alternative method of infant feeding. *Arch Child Dis* **71**: 365–369.
3. Lang S (1994) Cup-feeding: an alternative method. *Midwives Chron* **107**: 171–176.
4. Samuel P (1998) Cup feeding. Case histories of three term babies. *Pract Midwife* **1**: 33–35.
5. Meier P (1988) Bottle- and breast-feeding: effects on transcutaneous oxygen pressure and temperature in preterm infants. *Nurs Res* **37**: 36–40.
6. Meier P, Pugh E (1985) Breast-feeding behaviour of small preterm infants. *Am J Mat Child Nurs* **10**: 396–401.
7. Meier P, Anderson GC (1987) Responses of small preterm infants to bottle and breast feeding. *Am J Mat Child Nurs* **12**: 97–105.
8. Mead LJ, Chuffo R, Lawlor-Klean P et al (1992) Breastfeeding success with preterm quadruplets. *JOGNN* **21**: 79–85.
9. Whitelaw A, Heisterkamp G, Sleath K et al (1988) Skin to skin contact for very low birthweight infants and their mothers. *Arch Dis Child* **63**: 1377–1381.
10. Kelnar JH, Harvey D (1987) Nutrition. In: *The Sick Newborn Baby*, 2nd edn. Kelnar JH, Harvey D (eds). London: Baillière Tindall, pp. 134–159.
11. Hurst NM, Valentine CJ, Renfro L et al (1997) Skin-to-skin holding in the neonatal intensive care unit influences maternal milk volume. *J Perinatol* **17**: 213–217.
12. Salariya EM, Robertson CM (1993) Relationship between baby feeding types and patterns and gut transit time of meconium and the incidence of neonatal jaundice. *Midwifery* **9**: 235–242.
13. Schneider AP (1986) Breastmilk and jaundice in the newborn – a real entity. *JAMA* **225**: 3270–3274.
14. De Carvalho M, Klaus MH, Merkatz RB (1982) Frequency of breast-feeding and serum bilirubin. *Am J Dis Child* **136**: 737–738.
15. Auerbach KG, Gartner LM (1987) Breastfeeding and human milk: their association with jaundice in the neonate. *Clin Perinatol* **14**: 89–107.
16. Sullivan SA, Birch LL (1994) Infant dietary experience and acceptance of solid foods. *Pediatrics* **2**: 271–277.

17. Harris H (1994) *Matt and Mandy: A solution for breastfeeding attachment through co-bathing* [video]. Melbourne: Ace Graphics (http://www.acegraphics.com.au).
18. Koh THHG, Aynsley-Green A, Tarbit M (1988) Neuronal dysfunction during hypoglycaemia. *Arch Dis Child* **63**: 1353–1358.
19. World Health Organization (1997) *Hypoglycaemia of the Newborn. Review of the Literature.* WHO/CHD/97.1. Geneva: WHO.
20. Hawdon LM, Nugent M, Angel P (2000) Controversies regarding definition of neonatal hypoglycaemia: implications for neonatal nursing. *J Neonat Nurs* **6**: 169–171.
21. Hawdon JM, Ward-Platt MP, Aynsley-Green A (1992) Patterns of metabolic adaption in term and preterm infants in the first postnatal week. *Arch Dis Child* **67**: 357–365.
22. Hawdon JM, Ward-Platt MP, Aynsley-Green A (1993) Neonatal hypoglycaemia – blood glucose monitoring and baby feeding. *Midwifery* **9**: 3–6.
23. Cornblath M, Hawdon JM, Williams AF et al (2000) Controversies regarding definition of neonatal hypoglycaemia: suggested operational thresholds. *Pediatrics* **105**: 1141–1145.
24. Stanley CA, Baker L (1999) The causes of neonatal hypoglycaemia [editorial]. *N Engl J Med* **340**: 1200–1201.
25. Lawrence RA, Lawrence RM (1999) Breastfeeding the infant with a problem. In *Breastfeeding. A Guide for the Medical Profession,* 5th edn. New York: Mosby, pp. 443–507.
26. Smith K (1999) Breastfeeding the baby with gastroesophageal reflux. *LLLGB News* July/August: 13–14.
27. Morrison P (1999) HIV and infant feeding. To breastfeed or not to breastfeed: the dilemma of competing risks. Part 2. *Breastfeed Rev* **7**: 11–19.
28. Jeffrey BS, Mercer KG (2000) Pretoria pasteurisation: a potential method for the reduction of postnatal mother to child transmission of the human immunodeficiency virus. *J Trop Paediatr* **46**: 219–223.
29. McDougal JS (1990) Pasteurization of human breast milk and its effect on HIV infectivity. Presentation at the Annual Meeting of the Human Milk Banking Association of North America, Lexington, Kentucky, 15 October 1990.
30. John GC, Kneiss J (1996) Mother-to-child transmission of human immunodeficiency virus type 1. *Epidemiol Rev* **18**: 49–57.
31. Department of Health (1999) *HIV and Infant Feeding.* Guidance from the UK Chief Medical Officers' Expert Advisory on AIDS. London: DOH.
32. Coutsoudis A, Pillay E, Spooner E et al (1999) Influence of infant-feeding patterns on early mother-to-mother-transmission of HIV-1 in Durban, South Africa. A prospective cohort study. *Lancet* **354**: 471–476.

7

Alternative methods of feeding and breastfeeding

7.1 ALTERNATIVE AND SUPPLEMENTARY METHODS OF FEEDING

There are a number of alternative and supplementary feeding methods, which can be used in neonatal and paediatric units until breastfeeding is fully established. These include gastric tubes, direct expression, syringes and droppers, cup-feeding and spoons, the breastfeeding supplementer and bottle-feeding. Each method has its own unique role in feeding.

Some babies may need only one or two alternative feeding methods, while others may need to use several before they can fully breastfeed. The methods chosen should be part of a planned programme, taking the baby from admission through to discharge. In this way it is possible to break down into easy stages how breastfeeding will be achieved. Of course, not all mothers choose to breastfeed; some may choose to express their milk and give it by bottle, and others may choose to give formula milk. Whatever the goal is – and it may change during the baby's stay in a unit – there should still be a rational and logical progression to the methods chosen. Babies who are to be bottle-fed, for example, may also benefit from first of all learning how to cup-feed.

The oral feeding methods available to us are of two main types: baby-led, and carer-led. A baby-led method is one in which the baby can control the length of the feed and the amount taken. In the case of breastfeeding (with or without a breastfeeding supplementer) a baby can stop breastfeeding and detach himself from the breast; in cup-feeding, if a baby closes his mouth, milk will not be taken. These are both baby-led methods. All other methods, where milk is actively put into the baby's mouth and he has no control of the amount or the pace of the feed, are carer-led. These methods include use of the syringe or dropper, a spoon, or a bottle. A baby who is immature or ill may need to have control initially when orally feeding.

A good starting-point for any baby admitted to a neonatal or paediatric unit is to make a feeding plan. This should include all the possible methods of feeding that particular baby may require, in order to reach his eventual feeding method. It should be in order of physiological difficulty. An example is shown in Box 7.1. This feeding plan includes all the feeding options available, but can be tailored to the individual needs of a breast-fed or bottle-fed baby. It may or may not include a rough approximation of the time involved for each step. Its value is that the mother and those helping her have a simple, clear, written plan which shows appropriate methods of feeding that are likely to be used throughout the baby's stay. The plan also emphasizes the importance of skin and breast contact so that the baby can learn to breastfeed, alongside the other methods.

A mother should understand the reason why an alternative method of feeding is used, and what will be achieved by choosing one method over another. It is important that she knows how the methods used will enable her to achieve breastfeeding and how she can enhance her baby's feeding experiences. She also needs to know why certain devices should be avoided if possible, and how they can interfere with breast-feeding, or even cause her baby to refuse the breast. Nipple shields, dummies, bottles and teats, and finger-feeding all have a negative effect on a baby's ability to breastfeed – primarily because they do not follow the same physiological pathway as breastfeeding. At its simplest, a baby who opens his mouth only wide enough to accommodate these devices may not open his mouth wide enough to breastfeed successfully.

Breastfeeding is about anticipation. The smell of the areola stimulates the baby to open his mouth and attach to the breast. It may be important to encourage a baby to use his anticipatory responses, and a cup (for example) will do this. There is no such anticipation with bottle-feeding – the baby cannot smell the milk before he receives it.

Box 7.1 Example of a feeding plan. The layout is designed to emphasize the importance of skin and breast contact at every stage

Intravenous feeding	B
Nasal or oral gastric tube	R
Direct hand-expression	E
Syringe/dropper	A
Cup-feeding	S
Breastfeeding supplementer	T
Spoon-feeding	FEED

This chapter describes in detail the various feeding options available to the mother and to those who support her. Finger assessment of feeding is included, not because it is an alternative method of feeding, but because it can be a useful diagnostic method of assessing a baby's ability to suck and swallow effectively.

7.2 GASTRIC TUBES

◆ Gastric tubes (Fig. 7.1) are commonly used until a baby is able to take his feeds by mouth. The milk is delivered directly into

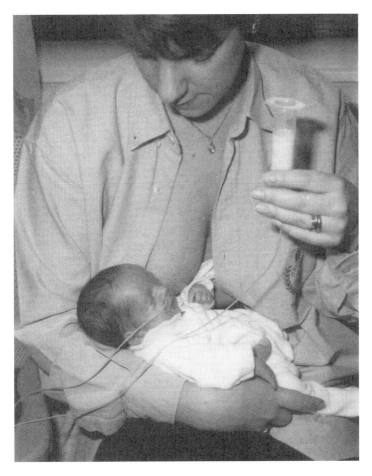

Figure 7.1 Gastric tube-feeding (photograph courtesy of the North Staffs Neonatal Unit).

the baby's stomach so he is not expected to either suck or swallow.

◆ Gastric tubes should only be used for as long as they are really needed. Digestion begins in the mouth, but gastric tubes bypass the lingual lipases at the back of the tongue, which help to break down milk fats. There is, however, a small amount of lipase activity in the stomach.

◆ The sensation of a gastric tube in the back of the throat may be unpleasant to the baby and inhibit him from using his suck and swallow reflexes properly.[1]

◆ There is some evidence to show that milk lipids can stick to the sides of the tubes, thus reducing the amount of fat (and energy) available to the baby.[2,3]

◆ A mother should be encouraged whenever possible to hold her baby next to her breast when he is being tube-fed. He can then smell and maybe lick or even attach to the breast, or just be comforted.

7.2.1 Breastfeeding and gastric tubes

Breastfeeding can usually be commenced when a baby has a gastric tube in place. The positioning of the baby is important. Breastfeeding with a nasogastric tube in place is easier than with an oral gastric tube. However, because the tube is in the nose it reduces the baby's nasal space and breathing capacity. It is important to make sure, in positioning and attachment, that the baby's nose is left as free as possible. The baby should be positioned with the tube-free nostril facing away from the nipple. Nasogastric tubes **should be avoided** if the baby has:

◆ nasal prong oxygen (reducing the space for a further nasal tube)
◆ breathing difficulties
◆ a cleft palate.

Orogastric tubes should be secured at the side of the mouth and cheek, to ensure free tongue movement. If tongue movement is restricted, it prevents the baby learning to extend his tongue or responding appropriately to the smell of the breast. This explains why orogastric tubes should not be secured over the chin, but by the side of the mouth (Figs 7.2 and 7.3).

Dental plates

If the baby has a dental plate, the underarm position may be the most practical. The mother should be aware that (unless she has a very protractile nipple or a very supple areola) the plate may prevent the baby taking much areola into his mouth, and the body may not have a very

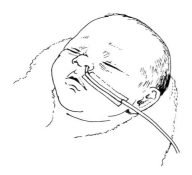

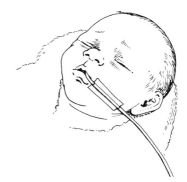

Figure 7.2 Securing a nasogastric tube.

Figure. 7.3 Securing an orogastric tube.

effective suck until the plate is removed. However, one can be proved wrong, and some very determined babies will suck strongly even with a plate in position. Gently expressing milk straight into the baby's mouth can be useful in this situation.

A dental plate with a gastric tube fitted into it should be removed as soon as the plate is no longer clinically required, so that the baby's palate is stimulated when he attaches to the breast. Dental plates, with a wire loop attached at the back of the plate to encourage swallowing, should be removed at the time of feeding, but left in place between feeds.

The following points are important to consider when a baby has a gastric tube in place and the mother wishes to breastfeed her baby.

Continuous and 1–2-hourly bolus tube-feeding

Milk may be given continuously by gastric tube until gastric tolerance and emptying are established. It is then usual for hourly bolus feeds to be commenced, with the feeds gradually becoming less frequent as the baby tolerates larger volumes. A gastric tube passed nasally or orally can be used. Some dental plates or obturators are designed to have an orogastric tube fitted into them. This secures the tube and ensures it will not easily become dislodged from the stomach. Oral tubes secured by the side of the mouth and cheek can be dislodged more easily by an active baby.

Milk feeds by continuous pump

Stop the pump during any attempt at breastfeeding. A pump is a convenient way to administer expressed breastmilk.

◆ The syringe should be positioned so that the nozzle is uppermost, thereby ensuring delivery of the richer milk first (which contains increased levels of fat and energy).
◆ To make certain the milk is kept as fresh as possible, and to reduce the chance of bacterial growth, put only 4 hours' worth of milk in the syringe at a time, and keep the remainder refrigerated or frozen until required.

Milk feeding by 1–2-hourly bolus tubes

If the mother is present when bolus milk feeds are given every 1–2 hours, encourage her to express some breastmilk on to her nipple for the baby to taste at the same time the milk is being given by tube. Position the baby so that if he shows signs of wanting to lick the breast or suckle, he can easily attach to the breast. It is preferable for the baby to experience sucking at the breast rather than on a dummy.

1. See what the baby will do at the breast before the next gastric feed is due.
2. On the initial occasion at the breast, direct expression will help a baby to become accustomed to the taste and smell of the milk, and attachment is made much simpler.
3. If a baby is unable to take a feed, or only takes a little, give the bolus via the tube while he is near or attached to the breast. Either the mother can gently express some milk for her baby to taste, or she can hold him close to the breast during the feed.
4. If a baby is able to take some good sucks from the breast, slightly delay the next bolus feed.
5. If the mother and hospital staff are happy that her baby has suckled well, *delay* the bolus feed for at least an hour or until he wants to feed again (whichever is sooner). While the baby is feeding every 1–2 hours, waiting will not harm a healthy, preterm baby and will greatly boost the mother's confidence.
6. If a tube is due to be changed, give the mother and her baby the opportunity to breastfeed without the tube in place.
7. If possible, begin to introduce a cup once a baby is on 2-hourly intermittent gastric tubes. Quite apart from the tactile experience, it is not stressful, and he can taste the milk and stimulate his tongue muscles and digestive juices, and generally enjoy his feed!

Three-hourly bolus gastric tube feeds

Initially these feeds may be given through a nasogastric tube left in place between feeds. Intermittent orogastric tube-feeding should be used as soon as possible so that the baby can also develop his ability to suck and swallow without any tubes in place. Breastfeeding should be attempted whenever possible, according to the baby's condition. Cup-feeding should be considered instead of tube-feeding whenever possible, but neither should be used if the baby can breastfeed.

When formula milk has to be used

There are several situations in which formula milk has to be used with expressed breastmilk. It is inevitable when a mother is not producing sufficient milk for her baby's needs, or where a low-birthweight formula is prescribed by the doctors. Human milk itself contains two lipases. One of these, bile salt stimulated lipase (BSSL), possibly aids improved fat absorption when a mixture of formula milk and the mother's own milk is given to a baby.[4] Therefore, any formula milk used should be mixed with some expressed breastmilk, even if this is a very small proportion of the total amount. Quite apart from the benefits to the baby, it helps the mother to feel her milk remains an important factor in her baby's progress. If human milk from a milk bank is available, it should be used instead of formula milk.

7.3 DIRECT EXPRESSION OF BREASTMILK

A mother can hand-express a little of her milk into her baby's mouth, or onto her nipple for him to taste, whenever he shows signs of wanting to suckle, or is held next to her breast (Fig. 7.4). Babies as young as 30 weeks (and sometimes as young as 27 or 28 weeks) can safely cope with a few drops of their mother's milk in this way. Direct expresson is useful for a baby who is about to be introduced to breastfeeding. It is a particularly useful technique for a baby who is preterm, weak or ill, because it requires little effort. It is also useful for a baby who initially fights at the breast or who is reluctant to suck. It gives the baby the taste of the milk, thereby stimulating the release of oral juices containing enzymes, which aid digestion. It also stimulates the movement of the jaw muscles and tongue, and encourages coordination of the suck and swallow reflex. There is nearly always a positive response in the baby. Even a baby treated with continuous positive airway pressure (CPAP) can lick milk from the breast while being held. Some babies on nasal CPAP are even able to suckle without any problem, although this should only be attempted if the baby shows that he is ready, by rooting or beginning to suck on the nipple (see if he will attach correctly), and has a stable heart and respiratory rate.

It is imperative, if this technique is used, that the mother knows how to hand-express correctly.

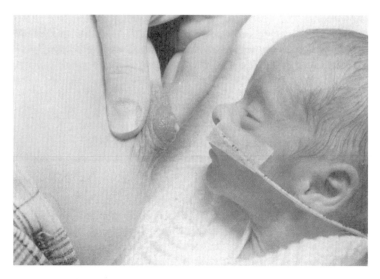

Figure 7.4 The direct expression of breastmilk (photograph courtesy of the North Staffs Neonatal Unit).

7.4 SYRINGES AND DROPPERS

A 1 mL; 2 mL or 5 mL syringe or a dropper can be used for small amounts of milk, such as colostrum, or occasionally to administer drugs. The lingual lipases are utilized, but the baby does not need to suck (though it is an advantage if he does). It is important that swallowing and breathing are well coordinated, because the baby cannot anticipate the milk until it is in his mouth. Neither is he in control of the amount of milk put into his mouth, thus there is an increased risk of its aspiration if his coordination is compromised. To avoid this, milk should never be put directly onto the baby's tongue, but instead into the cheek area or just under the tongue.

If the baby sucks on the syringe or dropper, a small amount of milk should be gently pushed into the baby's mouth as he is sucking, but not swallowing. This helps to prevent aspiration, which is always a danger when a baby is unable to pace his own intake. The baby should be held in a semi-sitting position, but should not be fed by syringe if he is lying flat on his back.

Droppers and syringes can also be used to drip milk onto the areola (Fig. 7.5), as described below:

1. A quantity of expressed breastmilk is put into a 10 mL or 20 mL syringe.

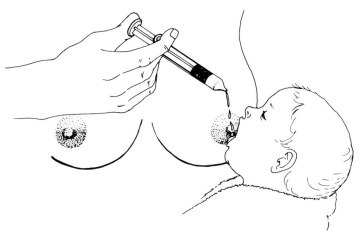

Figure 7.5 Using a syringe to encourage breastfeeding.

2. The baby is positioned at the breast, with his mouth close to the mother's nipple and areola.
3. A little breastmilk is squeezed onto the nipple area from the syringe.
4. The baby is encouraged to lick the milk from the nipple.
5. If he begins to open his mouth widely, his mother may attach him to the breast if possible. The milk from the syringe should be stopped at this point or just trickled on to the breast very slowly. If successful attachment is achieved, then use of the syringe can be discontinued.

This method may be useful for babies who refuse or are reluctant to attach to the breast, or for preterm babies who do not have the strength to suckle effectively, but are able to lick and swallow the milk trickled onto the breast. It may also help mothers whose let-down reflex is temporarily inhibited for whatever reason.

7.5 CUP-FEEDING

Babies are fed by cup in many different parts of the world. Cups are commonly used for preterm and low-birthweight babies.[5]
The cup provides a useful alternative to gastric tubes[6] and bottles[7,8] in a variety of different situations in which breastfeeding is not possible.[9–11] It is a simple, practical and safe method of feeding babies with a wide range of clinical problems. One of its primary advantages is that it is 'baby-led' not 'carer-led'. If a baby does not want to cup-feed, all he has to do is keep his mouth closed! Cup-feeding allows a baby to set the pace

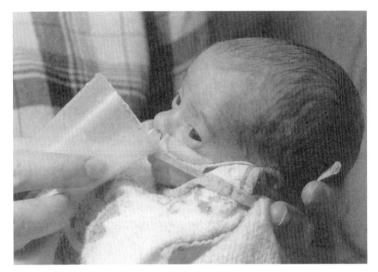

Figure 7.6 A preterm baby cup-feeding (photograph courtesy of the North Staffs Neonatal Unit).

at which he feeds, and therefore helps to protect his physical integrity. Physiologically it has several advantages, whether the baby eventually breastfeeds or bottlefeeds. It enables a baby to react in a totally appropriate way, for it encourages him to 'anticipate' the feed. The cup is open, so he can smell the milk (Fig. 7.6). The usual response, even from a baby of 29–30 weeks' gestation, is to extend his tongue and begin to search for the milk. He coats his tongue with milk and, by using rhythmic movements of his tongue and jaw, transports it to the back of his mouth, and swallows. The lingual lipases are utilized. Developing these movements is crucial, no matter how a baby is going to feed.

Because the baby does not need to suck, the cup is very useful with a baby who panics when he has a mouth full of breast, or is immature or weak, or when the mother's milk flow is very fast. If he can pace his own feed, both in time and quantity, he has time to 'enjoy' his milk. Many babies who require special care have unpleasant oral experiences: they may have been ventilated, have had frequent oral suction with catheters, and may have had oral or nasal tubes passed on a number of occasions or left in situ. It is important for a baby to have pleasant and enjoyable oral experiences. If, for whatever reason, breastfeeding is not possible, cup-feeding has many benefits, including giving the carer some indication of the baby's readiness to breastfeed.

Once a baby begins to dribble while cup-feeding, it is a sign that it is nearing the end of its physiological usefulness, and that the baby has reached a developmental milestone which needs to include active sucking – and he needs to breastfeed more often. Perhaps this is why cup-feeding is not as successful with healthy, term babies.

7.5.1 General reasons for using a cup

◆ To provide a positive oral experience for a baby.
◆ To provide an alternative method of feeding when a mother is not available to breastfeed her baby.
◆ To avoid any possibility of a baby having problems in breastfeeding as a result of being introduced to different sucking techniques.
◆ To reduce the need for nasal and oral gastric tubes.

Advantages of cup-feeding

◆ The baby paces his own intake in time and quantity.
◆ Little energy is used.
◆ It stimulates the development of the suck and swallow reflexes; coordination is also encouraged.
◆ Saliva and lingual lipases are stimulated, leading to a more efficient digestion of breastmilk.[12,13]
◆ Less fat is lost when milk is given with a cup rather than through a gastric tube.
◆ Eye contact is encouraged between the baby and the person giving the feed.
◆ The baby has to be held closely and securely for the feed.
◆ It is a very easy method of feeding.

Disadvantages of cup-feeding

◆ Term babies tend to dribble!
◆ Term, healthy babies can become addicted to the cup if they cannot go to the breast regularly.
◆ It is so easy for health professionals to use a cup, that occasionally it is used when it may be more appropriate to try the baby at the mother's breast.
◆ If the cup is held too tightly in contact with the baby's lips or gums, the skin can be blistered or broken. This is not common, but can occur if the cup has a sharp rim or is not held in a relaxed manner.

A cup should not replace breastfeeding without very good reason.

7.5.2 When and how to use a cup

A cup should be used when an alternative to the gastric tube is required. This may be because the baby is not able to feed from the breast or from a bottle (if he is to be formula-fed), or because the baby is preterm or sick, or the mother is not present on the unit to breastfeed.

The preterm baby

A cup can be safely used to feed a healthy, preterm baby from approximately 30 weeks' gestation, or when a baby shows signs that he is becoming more active orally. It is possible for a baby to cup-feed before he is able to breastfeed efficiently. However, it should **never** be used instead of a breastfeed, i.e. where the baby is able to satisfy all or part of his nutritional needs from the breast. Feeding from the breast still remains the safest way for a baby to be fed,[14] including a baby born preterm. Ideally cup-feeding and learning to breastfeed should take place at the same time.

A cup may be appropriate when:

◆ a preterm baby is wide awake and restless at feed times
◆ a baby shows signs of wanting to suck, e.g. sucking on his fist
◆ a baby is not satisfied by tube feeds and is restless after the feed
◆ a baby is not yet able to feed directly from the breast, or has only enough energy to satisfy part of his total nutritional needs at the breast.

The majority of preterm babies receive their milk through nasal or oral gastric tubes. Cup-feeding may be commenced when bolus tube feeds every 2–3 hours are introduced or established. It is not usually appropriate while continuous or hourly bolus feeds are required, or where there is evidence that the baby is not absorbing his milk feeds. There is some evidence to suggest that gastric tubes delay the development of the suck and swallow coordination in babies.[1] This is a particularly important factor to consider when cup-feeding preterm babies, for one of its purposes is to encourage the development of these reflexes and their coordination. It is vital, therefore, that gastric tubes are removed as soon as possible. However, it must be left to the discretion of the carer whether it is possible or appropriate to remove a gastric tube prior to a cup feed.

A preterm baby having only one or two feeds a day by any alternative method should have the tube left in place. When three or more feeds are given by a method other than a gastric tube, the tube should be removed, initially to see how well the baby does without it. The tube may have to be replaced, and it is important for parents to be aware of this possibility. At this stage, intermittent use of an oral tube may be more appropriate.

When the baby is initially being introduced to the breast and having the occasional cup feed as well, it may be a useful compromise to give the baby gastric tube feeds overnight and alternate the breast with a cup during the day. If supplementary feeds are still required, these can be given after the breastfeed by cup. Otherwise the cup should be used instead of the tube when the baby is able to go to the breast successfully on three or more occasions a day. The gastric tube should be removed at this time, but should be replaced if there is any concern over the baby's weight gain.

When preterm babies cup-feed, they are often observed to 'lap', by protruding their tongue and taking an amount of milk on their tongue, in this way they are also learning to cope with small boluses of milk in their mouths. As they mature, they begin to 'sip' the milk. It is normal for a range of facial expressions to be seen after stimulation of the lips with the cup. At no time should cup-feeding cause distress to a baby. If it does, it may be that either the baby is being held in an inappropriate position, e.g. semi-reclining, or the cup is being placed too far forward on the upper lip or pressing on the lower lip or gums. It may also indicate that milk is being tipped into the baby's mouth, causing him to panic.

The term baby

Cup-feeding is *not* appropriate for a term, healthy baby who can maintain his nutritive needs at the breast. It may, however, be useful if the mother has had a caesarean section or is ill following delivery, or if the baby requires any oral drugs. Very occasionally cup-feeding may also help a term baby who has become used to a bottle teat or dummy and is having difficulty correctly attaching to the breast. In this case, when repeated attempts to attach him to the breast have failed and the mother feels a bottle is her only choice, a cup can be used for up to 24 hours (using the mother's expressed breastmilk) before trying to establish breastfeeding again. It may help to use a position for breastfeeding which is different to the one used previously. Special attention should be paid to the attachment of the baby. If a gastric tube has been used to feed him on a neonatal or paediatric unit, then progression to cup-feeding should follow the same guidelines as for the preterm baby. Some term babies refuse cup-feeding altogether, while other term babies who become used to cup-feeding may become addicted to a cup and have to be weaned from it. Where a cup is used with a term, healthy or ill baby, it is important to let the baby feed as often as possible at the breast to avoid this happening.

7.5.3 The baby with special requirements

Much of what has already been written applies in the situation of a baby with special requirements. Cup-feeding in the following two situations is particularly useful.

The baby with a cleft lip and/or cleft palate

Cup-feeding should be used if there is a possibility that the baby will be able to breastfeed. It can be used in the period during which establishment of breastfeeding is taking place. It is helpful to give an initial small amount by cup so that the baby is less frustrated initially at the breast. The direct expression of breastmilk is also very important in establishing breastfeeding with these babies. A cup can be used for a unilateral or bilateral cleft lip and palate.[15]

The baby who cannot suck effectively

Cup-feeding has a particularly important role in the care of babies unable to feed from either the breast or a bottle. After it has been established that the baby's ability to suck from the nipple or teat is compromised but the baby is able to swallow without difficulty, try cup-feeding, particularly if the only alternative is gastric tube-feeding for weeks or even months.

The baby laps or sips the milk initially from a cup, an action that is frequently possible with babies who have neurological problems. The baby's ability to suck may develop slowly and gradually along with his ability to coordinate his suck – swallow and breathing reflexes. This may take from a few days to several months. Cup-feeding encourages the coordinated movement of the tongue and muscles of the mouth, while also allowing the baby to enjoy his feeds. This may be very important in the future of such a baby. Early feeding experiences are often of great importance, particularly if the child can associate feeding with pleasant experiences. Passing gastric tubes over long periods can be a nerve-racking experience for nursing staff, parents and for the child. Parents can safely cup-feed a baby at home.

If the mother wishes to breastfeed her baby, encourage skin-to-skin contact, and the expression of milk onto her nipples or into her baby's mouth, which will help to stimulate his tongue movement. Gently stroking the baby's lips will also stimulate him to open his mouth. A mother may find these simple strategies more rewarding than giving her baby a dummy, because although the baby may be able to suck on a dummy, the technique he adopts may not be correct for successful nutritive sucking at the breast. If it is necessary to assess the baby's sucking ability, it is preferable to use a clean finger. As time passes, the baby may be able to suck efficiently, not only on a dummy, but may also be able to breastfeed or bottle-feed successfully. Patience and persever-ance are certainly needed.

7.5.4 How much should the baby take?

The amount to be taken by the baby will depend upon a number of factors:

1. Initially a preterm baby may only take a small amount from the cup, maybe 5–10 mL. This is particularly the case for an immature baby. It is worth giving him the opportunity of cup-feeding at least once a day.

He should then be given the rest of his feed by gastric tube. The baby's response is usually very positive.

2. Once the baby is taking two or more cup feeds a day, unless a very small amount has been taken and there is good reason, do not 'top him up' – wait until the baby wants more milk, or the next feed. Babies whatever their gestational age may want very little milk at one feed and a large volume at the next. It is the 24-hour total that is important.

3. If the baby has taken at least half of his requirement at a particular feed it is preferable to wait until he next wants more milk. If the baby is not yet waking to demand his feeds and is having 2-hourly feeds, wait till the next feed is due. If he is on 3-hourly feeds, also wait until the next feed is due (if this is possible) or for at least an hour before 'topping up', particularly if a gastric tube has to be passed.

4. In the case of a baby who is capable of breastfeeding but not yet able to satisfy all his needs from the breast, allow him to have more milk from a cup after the feed. The amount he takes should not be regulated, unless the baby is fluid-restricted or the breastfeed was very short.

5. If a preterm (or term) baby initially 'fights' at the breast and direct expression does not help, give a small amount of milk by cup before the breastfeed continues, to settle him.

7.5.5 Method of cup-feeding

The method of cup-feeding is the same for any baby, regardless of gestational age. It is easy to feed a baby with a cup, but as with any alternative method of feeding, there are dangers if it is not done properly. If milk is poured into a baby's mouth there is a risk of aspiration.[16] To avoid this, the method of feeding described below should be followed. It is a good idea to let a mother observe one or two cup feeds being given by nursing staff, before she uses a cup herself.[10,17] Give her written instructions as well, emphasizing the need for the baby to be sitting in a semi-upright position and the cup to be held at the lips only.

What to use in hospital

A 60 mL medicine measure makes an ideal cup, as long as the rim is not too sharp. These can easily be sent to the hospital's sterilizing unit. Cups with lids and with a rounded rim are available; the advantage of these is that a mother can express milk straight into the cup, which can then be put into a freezer or a refrigerator.

What to use at home

An eggcup can be used as long as it has a reasonably thin, rounded rim. It should be made in one piece so that bacteria cannot contaminate the milk from any joins. Another useful 'cup' is the hard plastic cover for a teat in a bottle set, as long as the rim is rounded and smooth. Some commercially available hand-pump sets may include cups rather than bottles.

Method for feeding

1. Wrap the baby securely, to prevent his hands knocking the cup. Use a terry nappy placed under his chin. (This can be weighed both prior to and after the feed, if necessary – for dribble factor!)
2. Support the baby in a semi-upright sitting position (Fig. 7.7).
3. If possible have the cup at least half-full for the beginning of the feed. (This is particularly helpful for the person learning the technique, so that milk is not poured into the baby's mouth.)
4. The cup should be tipped so the milk is just touching the baby's lips. **Do not pour milk into the baby's mouth**.
5. Direct the rim of the cup towards the corners of the upper lip and gums, with it gently or touching or resting on the baby's lower lip. Do not apply pressure to the lower lip.
6. Leave the cup in the correct position during the feed. Do not keep removing it when the baby stops drinking. It is important to let the baby pace his own intake in his own time.

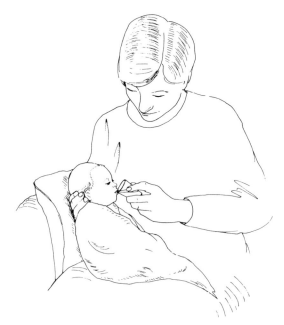

Figure 7.7 The position to hold a baby for cup-feeding.

Type of milk to use

Expressed breastmilk is the ideal milk to use. However, formula milk can also be given by cup. Always shake the bottle containing expressed milk to ensure a more even distribution of the milk fat.

The bondla or palladai

Cups to feed babies have existed for centuries and are common in many parts of the world. In the Indian subcontinent a cup is used that has a long, pointed lip. This cup is known as a *palladai* or *bondla*.[17,18] Small amounts of milk are trickled into the front of the baby's mouth. This is commonly used in hospitals to feed expressed breastmilk to small babies.

7.6 SPOONS

Using a spoon is a carer-led feeding method. A small amount of milk can either be put into the baby's mouth,[17,18] or the baby can lap the milk out of the spoon. If a baby is preterm, ill or weak, it is better not to put the milk directly into the baby's mouth but to let him take the milk he wants

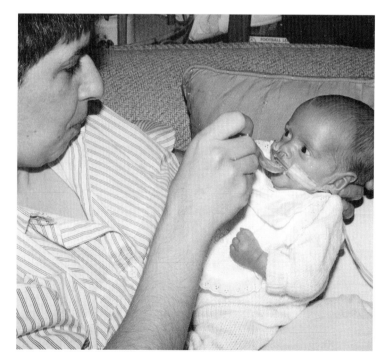

Figure 7.8 Spoon-feeding.

by lapping or sipping. If milk is put into the baby's mouth it should be put just inside the mouth or under the tongue. Some mothers find using a spoon rather awkward,[19] with moderate amounts of spillage possible.

One of the main disadvantages for babies in a neonatal unit of spoon-feeding is that the baby is not in control of the size of the bolus of milk or the pace of the feeds; however, it is ideal to use when the baby starts on semi-solids (Fig. 7.8).

7.7 THE BREASTFEEDING SUPPLEMENTER

The breastfeeding supplementer can be used to help a baby feed from the breast when the mother is experiencing difficulty with her milk supply.[19] It enables a mother to stimulate her milk production in a natural and satisfying way. (Fig. 7.9). It avoids the need to use other methods of feeding and is particularly useful if a baby has a cleft lip and palate, or is

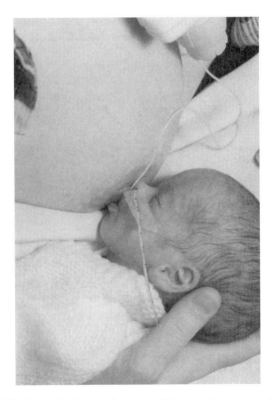

Figure 7.9 The breastfeeding supplementer (photograph courtesy of the North Staffs Neonatal Unit).

weak, or the mother's milk flow is slow. It has many of the advantages of breastfeeding, and is a method that is probably very underused in view of its advantages. It should be considered in the following situations:

◆ Situations affecting the mother:
  – a genuinely low milk production
  – persistently insufficient milk supply
  – breast surgery
  – relactation (after established breastfeeding, or to initiate lactation in the case of adoption).
◆ Situations affecting the baby:
  – a weak suck, due to prematurity
  – a weak suck, due to neurological damage
  – a weak suck, due to a chromosomal abnormality, e.g. Down's syndrome
  – a cross baby who will not attach to the breast.

7.7.1 Method

It is important to attach the breastfeeding supplementer to the breast correctly.

1. Fill the container with the required amount of milk.
2. Make sure the lid is on securely.
3. Hang the container around the neck, so that it hangs between the breasts in a position level with the nipples or just above.
4. Attach the tubes to the nipples. Each tube should be secured in position on the top of the breasts, with the tip of each tube protruding very slightly over the end of each nipple. The tape used to secure the tubes should be placed above the areola.
5. Position the baby and attach to the breast in the normal way.

If the supplementer has a valve system it may be necessary to release the valve at this point so that the milk flows freely as the baby suckles.

It is important to choose the correct size tubing for the baby: some designs come with a variety of different tube sizes, from the equivalent of a 0.4 to a 0.8 gauge feeding tube. It is useful to begin with the largest size. If the baby is to be breastfed in the future without the supplementer, then the narrower tubes can be gradually introduced, so that less milk is obtained from the supplementer, and more is taken from the mother. It is also important to control the milk flow as appropriate. As the baby's suck grows stronger and/or the mother's milk flow increases, so the milk flow from the breastfeeding supplementer should be lessened. Some models have a series of notches in the lid into which the tube can be fixed. These are used to slow or reduce the milk flow or completely stop it.

The position of the tubes at the nipple may also need to be adjusted as the need for the breastfeeding supplementer lessens, as some babies can and do become addicted to the tube! The tube can gradually be moved around the areola until it is on the underside; it can then be withdrawn completely. Alternatively, the tube can be attached further up the breast until it is no longer in the baby's mouth.

The baby is able to take what he wants from the mother, in addition to the milk in the breastfeeding supplementer. It is important not to supplement the baby after the feed on the evidence of what has been taken from the visible milk supply. It is better to rely on how the mother feels:

◆ Do her breasts feel softer?
◆ Is the baby obviously satisfied?
◆ Does the baby settle well after the feed?
◆ Can you hear/see the baby swallow?

7.7.2 How to make a breastfeeding supplementer

A simple breastfeeding supplementer can be made very easily (Fig. 7.10). Use a cup or bottle of milk, with the end of a size 0.4 or 0.6 feeding tube placed in the milk, and the tip of the tube secured just above the mother's areola, with the tip very slightly over the end of the nipple (as previously described). The milk is then obtained when the baby begins to feed from the breast.

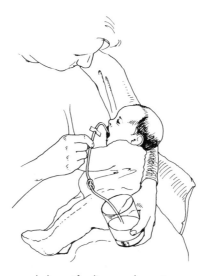

Figure 7.10 A home made breastfeeding supplementer.

7.7.3 Long-term use of the breastfeeding supplementer

A mother who is not able to produce sufficient of her own milk for her baby can still breastfeed using a breastfeeding supplementer. She may find having at least three supplementers will be useful. She can wear one of them under her clothes, so that she is always ready for when her baby wishes to breastfeed. The milk will be at the right temperature when the baby suckles. The remaining two supplementers can be kept in the refrigerator until required. If formula milk is used it can be made up in the mornings so that there is always milk available. Human milk from a milk bank can also be used. The milk should then be used preferably within 4–6 hours once it is at body temperature.

7.8 FINGER ASSESSMENT OF FEEDING

Finger assessment is a simple and effective diagnostic method of assessing a baby's ability to suck and swallow efficiently. It allows assessment of tongue movement and the baby's ability to cope with milk boluses. However, it should only be used for this purpose where conventional feeding methods continually fail.

Note the movement of the tongue. It should move in a rhythmical way from the front to the back and form a furrow around the finger (or breast/nipple). An uncoordinated tongue may be haphazard in its movement, creating pressure on parts of the palate that are inappropriate for sucking or for eliciting the swallow reflex. Where this happens, cup-feeding may help to correct the problem. Gentle agitation with the tip of the finger on the junction of the hard and soft palate should cause a swallow response. Milk should not be given unless a swallow reflex is present.

Finger assessment may be useful when a baby is admitted for 'poor feeding' and does not appear to improve with any conventional method of feeding.

The method is as follows:

1. Wash hands carefully.
2. Fill a cup with the amount of milk the baby is due to have.
3. Place one end of a size 0.4 or 0.6 gastric tube on the pad of the index finger, the other in the cup of milk.
4. Fix the tube at the first joint of the finger with tape (Fig. 7.11).
5. At the same time as putting your finger in the baby's mouth, with the pad directed towards the hard palate, hold the cup slightly higher than the baby so that as soon as he begins to suck, the milk will flow. Once the milk is in the tube, put the cup in a convenient place.

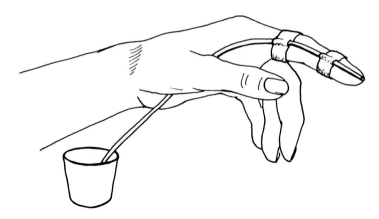

Figure 7.11 The position of a feeding tube for finger assessment of feeding.

Finger feeding is a technique used in some parts of the world, primarily to help babies who do not attach to the breast after birth[20] for breast refusal, and as a temporary feeding method for mothers with sore nipples.[21] However, the sucking technique used by the baby is very similar to the technique of bottle-feeding. It should, therefore, be used with extreme caution if breastfeeding is the desired outcome.

7.9 THE BOTTLE

It is better to avoid using bottles altogether if a baby is to be breastfed. When the situation arises in hospital where an alternative oral method of feeding or supplementation is required, health professionals can use a cup[22] or a spoon, and a mother may additionally use a breastfeeding supplementer or a syringe.

However, if it is the wish of a mother to go home breast- and bottle-feeding, it is important to find out why exclusive breastfeeding is not possible. For example, perhaps the mother is going back to work, and believes she must get her baby used to a bottle; perhaps she feels family pressure to share the baby's feeding; or perhaps she feels apprehensive at the idea of the baby being entirely dependent on her. Whatever the reason, make sure the mother is aware that alternatives to the bottle do exist and can be used safely. If she is returning to work, it is worth talking through the options: such as finding a childminder near her workplace so that she can breastfeed during the day, or considering crèche facilities. If more mothers ask for these facilities, the more likely they are to be made available.

If a mother is certain that she wishes to introduce bottles, find out if expressed breastmilk or formula milk is to be used. If she wishes to use expressed breastmilk she needs to be confident in her skill of expressing and know how to hand-express. Even if she does not intend to use this method, it can be useful if her hand or electric pump fails. She also needs to know how to store the milk safely. If the mother plans to use formula milk, she should be aware that her own milk supply may diminish, if she does not express regularly and has insufficient breast stimulation. Some babies will also develop a preference for either the breast or the bottle, so it is important that a baby is established at the breast before a bottle (or a dummy) is introduced.

If a mother is having problems with breastfeeding that do not appear to respond to help, she should be encouraged to continue breastfeeding whenever possible, even if a bottle is introduced. She should not feel under pressure to feed only by bottle or only by breast, particularly if this results in breastfeeding being abandoned unnecessarily. It is possible for some babies to feed by both methods – and it is better to have some breastfeeds than none at all. Explain the situation to the mother's health visitor or community midwife. Also encourage the mother to contact her local Breastfeeding Network, National Childbirth Trust, La Leche League or Association of Breastfeeding Mothers breastfeeding counsellor to ensure she has consistent support and information after discharge (see appendix).

7.9.1 Preterm babies and bottle-feeding

Preterm babies who are to be breastfed should not be given bottles. It is important they learn to breastfeed without being confused by using another sucking pattern.

7.9.2 Bottle teats, dummies and the vulnerable baby

Permission (preferably written) should be obtained from the parents before a bottle or dummy is given to any baby who is to be breastfed.

If a baby is to be bottle-fed, he can be given a dummy quite safely, without the danger of teaching an inappropriate feeding technique – although it is worth remembering that allergy to latex is increasing and is associated with use of teats and dummies. Both dummies and nipple shields encourage the same pattern of sucking movements as bottle teats, because they are static in the mouth, unlike the breast which is softer and more pliable.

If a breastfed baby is admitted to the unit with feeding problems, a dummy may simply encourage an inappropriate sucking action or reinforce incorrect tongue movements, thus making the problem worse.

For mothers of babies with difficulties in feeding directly from the breast (such as cleft lip and/or palate), expressed breastmilk can be given by bottle, if breastfeeding is not considered possible (and the mother wants to use this method of feeding), using special teats, which allow the milk flow to be regulated.

7.10 MIXED BREASTFEEDING AND BOTTLE-FEEDING

Some babies are able to feed from both the breast and bottle without any apparent difficulty. When establishment of breastfeeding has taken place before the introduction to a bottle or dummy, a baby appears less likely to have problems with the two different sucking techniques. However, it is impossible to know which babies will manage the two methods of feeding without any problems and which babies will go on to refuse to breastfeed or bottle-feed. A period of time, preferably, at least 4–6 weeks, should be allowed to elapse before introducing a bottle to a clinically well baby, born at term. The period of time suggested is arbitrary but is long enough to allow a baby to become well established at the breast first. It is ideal to delay introducing a bottle to a preterm baby until he has reached at least 37 weeks' post-conception age or is well established at the breast, which may be later or earlier than 37 weeks. Preterm babies appear to be more susceptible than term babies to problems of adapting to different techniques of sucking.[23] One of the main dangers of introducing bottles, from the mother's point of view, is that her milk production may begin to decrease in the absence of maximum stimulation of the breasts, particularly in the first 6 weeks after birth.

Gestational age at birth and level of maturity at the time of the introduction of oral feeding may substantially influence whether a baby can feed successfully by both breast and bottle. Some term babies appear to develop a preference for a bottle teat. They are capable of feeding from either and can distinguish between the different techniques for suckling at the breast or sucking on a bottle teat. They may eventually prefer one to the other. Some preterm babies appear to become genuinely confused about how to feed from the breast or from a bottle teat, especially if they are introduced to different feeding techniques before breastfeeding has been established. Similarly, a baby who is ill at birth or shortly afterwards, regardless of gestational age, and who is able to feed orally, may use only one method of feeding and refuse the other method. If, for example, bottle-feeding has been the dominant method of feeding, then the baby may reject breastfeeding, and vice versa. A term baby who is ill at birth or becomes ill in the early postnatal period may temporarily lose the mature coordination of the suck, swallow and breathing reflexes necessary for effective nutritive feeding. This baby may relapse into feeding in the way he finds the most familiar.

There is no evidence to show that different-shaped teats make it easier for a baby to adapt to breastfeeding. Where mothers want to have the opportunity to feed with both methods, the use of different teats, which make the baby open his mouth wider or remove the milk using compression, should be examined. These teats may also have some advantages for the exclusively bottle-fed baby.

REFERENCES

1. Kelnar JH, Harvey D (1987) Delay of development of suck reflex in infants. In: *The Sick Newborn Baby*, 2nd edn. Kelnar JH, Harvey D (eds). London: Baillière Tindall, pp. 134–159.
2. Martenez FE, Desai ID, Davidson AGF et al (1987) Ultrasound homogenization of expressed human milk to prevent fat loss during tube feeding. *J Pediatr Gastroenterol Nutri* **6**: 593–597.
3. Brennan-Bohm M, Carlson GE, Meier et al (1994) Caloric loss from expressed mother's milk during continuous gavage infusion. *Neonat Network* **13**: 27–32.
4. Hamosh M, Bitman J, Fink CS et al (1985) Lipid composition of preterm human milk and its digestion by the infant. In: *Composition and Physiological Properties of Human Milk*. Schaub J (ed.). Oxford: Elsevier, pp. 153–162.
5. BFHI (1999). *Baby-Friendly hospital Initiative Newsletter* May/June 1999 [This newsletter concentrates on cupfeeding]. New York: UNICEF.
6. Giroux JD, Sizun J, Alix D (1991) L'alimentation a la tasse chez le nouveau-né. *Arch Fr Pediatr* **48**: 737–740.
7. Gupta A, Khanna K, Chattree S (1999) Cup feeding: an alternative to bottle feeding in a neonatal intensive care unit. *J Trop Paediatr* **45**: 108–110.
8. Howard CR, de Blieck EA, ten Hoopen CB et al (1999) Physiological stability of newborns during cup- and bottle feeding. *Pediatrics* **104**: 1204–1206.
9. Lang S, Lawrence CJ, L'E Orme R (1994) Cup feeding: an alternative method of infant feeding. *Arch Child Dis* **71**: 365–369.
10. Lang S (1994) Cup-feeding: an alternative method. *Midwives Chron* **107**: 171–176.
11. Armstrong HC (1998) Techniques of feeding infants: the case for cup feeding. *Research in Action* No. 8. New York: UNICEF, Nutrition Section, pp. 1–6.
12. Smith LJ (1986) Neonatal fat digestion and lingual lipase. *Acta Paediatr Scand* **75**: 913–918.
13. Lebenthal E, Heitlinger L, Milla PJ (1988) Prenatal and perinatal development of the gastrointestinal tract. In: *Harries Paediatric Gastroenterology*, 2nd edn. Milla PJ, Muller DPR (eds). Edinburgh: Churchill Livingstone, pp. 3–29.
14. Freer Y (1999) A comparison of breast and cup feeding in preterm infants: effect on physiological parameters. *J Neonat Nurs* **5**: 16–21.
15. Samuel P (1998) Cup feeding. Case histories of three term babies. *Pract Midwife* **1**: 33–35.
16. Thorley V (1997) Cup-feeding: problems created by incorrect use. *J Hum Lact* **13**: 54–55.

17. Nyqvist KH, Strandell E (1999) A cup feeding protocol for neonates: evaluation of nurses' and parents' use of two cups. *J Pediatr Nurs* **5**: 31–36.
18. Nair PMC, Narang A, Mahajan R et al (1994) Spoon feeds – an alternative to bottle feeding. *Indian Pediatr* **31**: 1566–1567.
19. Kumar H, Singhal PK, Singh S et al (1989) Spoon vs bottle: evaluation of milk feeding in young infants. *Indian Pediatr* **26**: 11–17.
20. Corbett M (2000) *Malnutrition in the infant less than 6 months: use of supplemental suckling technique.* Department of Medicine and Therapeutics, Foresterhill, Aberdeen.
21. Auerbach KG, Riordan J, Countryman BA (1993) The breastfeeding process. In: *Breastfeeding and Human Lactation.* Riordan J, Auerbach KG (eds). London: Jones & Bartlett, pp. 221–222.
22. Newman J (1990) Breastfeeding problems associated with the early introduction of bottles and pacifiers. *J Hum Lact* **6**: 59–63.
23. Armstrong H (1986) *Are Feeding Bottles Ever Needed?* Breastfeeding Briefs. Geneva: Infant Feeding Association.

Breastfeeding and common drugs

8.1 BREASTFEEDING AND DRUGS

Always ask a mother who is breastfeeding or who intends to breastfeed if she is taking any medicines. There is an extensive list in the *British National Formulary* on drugs and breastfeeding (a copy of this is available in all hospital clinical areas), the World Health Organization's *Annex on Breastfeeding and Maternal Medication Recommendations for Drugs in the Essential Drugs List* and in *Medications and Mothers' Milk*.[1-3] This last book is published each year and is a comprehensive text, covering over 750 drugs. At least one of these books should be consulted whenever there is any doubt over a drug given to a lactating mother.

Breastmilk is generally free from contamination, although certain drugs and other substances can be passed into the milk from the mother's bloodstream. It is important, therefore, to make sure that medicines or remedies from any source are compatible with breastfeeding. Ask the mother about any treatments she is having that may be based on homeopathy, aromatherapy or other less obvious practices. Many of these remedies are now bought 'over the counter' without any consultation with a specialist. It is quite possible, if a mother is experiencing a problem with her milk supply or the baby is refusing her breast, that she may be taking some form of medicine without realizing that it could have a negative effect on her lactation in some way – even if it only makes the milk less palatable to her baby! Remember that:

- Mothers should have no drugs during the nursing period unless prescribed by a doctor.
- The mother must remember to inform her doctor that she is breastfeeding if she needs any medication during this period.
  A prepared form, on which her doctor could write down any drugs the mother is prescribed, and which could be kept with her baby's

notes, would be useful, particularly if the medication is not well known.

◆ Ask the mother if she is on any drugs and if so, what they are. Check for yourself if it is safe for her to take them while breastfeeding. Check with a doctor on the unit or with the pharmacy, if you are unsure or worried.

8.1.1 Some common drugs to avoid

The combined contraceptive pill

The combined contraceptive pill, containing oestrogen and progesterone, should be avoided during lactation. Products containing oestrogen are known to cause significant reductions in milk volume – one study found this to be by as much as 40%.[4,5] Therefore, if low milk supply suddenly becomes a problem at around 6 weeks, check whether a mother has begun taking the combined pill. It is important, if she has resumed taking oral contraception, to ensure she is taking a progestogen-only pill ('mini-pill'). However, this is not without its drawbacks either, for evidence suggests that progestogens can cause a reduction in the fat content of breastmilk.[4]

Caffeine

Although tea, coffee and Coca-Cola are not drugs in the accepted sense, caffeine is! Caffeine can pass into breastmilk, but this does not usually cause problems. However, if a mother is accustomed to drinking several cups of strong coffee (six to eight) per day, it may cause restlessness in her baby. If a mother cannot completely give up drinks containing caffeine, advise her to have her drink shortly after breastfeeding and, if possible, to drink weaker coffee or tea. Using decaffeinated brands of coffee, tea or soft drinks will lessen, but not totally eliminate, her caffeine consumption.

Nicotine

Smoking should be discontinued if at all possible.[6,7] Nicotine is potentially hazardous to a baby in much the same way as it is to children and adults. Where a mother is unable to give up cigarettes, she should smoke after breastfeeding, not before. Smoking can, through vasoconstriction, considerably diminish the milk supply. Encourage the mother and her partner to smoke less. Passive intake of smoke is also hazardous and should be avoided whenever possible. It is particularly hazardous for a baby to sleep with his parents if they are smokers.

8.2 BREASTFEEDING AND MATERNAL MEDICATION

The following information gives a brief outline, based on the advice of the World Health Organization, on drugs prescribed to a mother and breastfeeding.[2]

8.2.1 Medication with contraindications to breastfeeding

◆ Anticancer drugs.
◆ Radioactive substances (in this case breastfeeding may be stopped for a temporary period only). Express and discard the milk until breastfeeding can be resumed.

8.2.2 Medication with which breastfeeding can be continued

Psychiatric drugs and anticonvulsants – **side-effects are possible** and the baby should be monitored for drowsiness.
Use an alternative to the following drugs if possible:

◆ chloramphenicol
◆ tetracyclines
◆ metronidazole
◆ quinolone antibiotics (e.g. ciprofloxacin).

The following drugs may **decrease the milk supply**, therefore alternatives should be used whenever possible:

◆ oestrogen
◆ thiazide diuretics
◆ ergometrine.

The baby should be **monitored for jaundice** if the following drugs are taken by the mother:

◆ sulfonamides
◆ co-trimoxazole (trimethoprim and sulfamethoxazole)
◆ Fansidar (pyrimethamine with sulfadoxine)
◆ dapsone.

The following drugs are **safe in normally prescribed dosages**; however, the **baby should be monitored** when they are taken by the mother:

◆ analgesics: short courses of paracetamol, acetylsalicylic acid, ibuprofen and occasional doses of morphine and pethidine

◆ antibiotics: penicillin, ampicillin, cloxacillin, erythromycin
◆ antihistamines
◆ antacids
◆ digoxin
◆ insulin
◆ bronchodilators (e.g. salbutamol)
◆ corticosteroids
◆ anthelmintics
◆ chloroquine
◆ antituberculous drugs.

Nutritional supplements of iron, iodine and vitamins can also be taken in the prescribed dosages.
Whenever possible, drugs should be avoided during the breast-feeding period.

REFERENCES

1. *British National Formulary* [published twice-yearly]. London: British Medical Association/Royal Pharmaceutical Society.
2. World Health Organization (1993) *Annex on Breastfeeding and Maternal Medication Recommendations for Drugs in the Essential Drugs List.* Geneva: WHO.
3. Hale T (2000) *Medications and Mothers' Milk,* 9th edn. Amarillo: Pharmasoft Medical Publishing.
4. Tankeyoon M, Dusitsin N, Chalapati S et al (1984) Effects of hormonal contraception on milk volume and infant growth. *Contraception* **30**: 505–522.
5. World Health Organization (1989) Infant feeding: the physiological basis. *WHO Bull* **67** (suppl.): 41–54.
6. Carlson DE (1988) Maternal diseases associated with intra-uterine growth retardation. *Perinatology* **12**: 17–22.
7. Fox H (1991) A contemporary view of the human placenta. *Midwifery* **17**: 31–39.

Recommendations for the support of breastfeeding

9.1 RECOMMENDATIONS FOR THE SUPPORT OF BREASTFEEDING ON A NEONATAL OR SPECIALIST PAEDIATRIC UNIT

Lactation management should have an important place in the overall plan of care within a neonatal or similar specialist unit. Skin contact between a mother and her baby, the non-verbal communication which is another side of breastfeeding, the continuation of the symbiotic relationship started in the womb and the act of nurturing, need to be protected. It may well be that the acute needs of a baby are uppermost in the minds of those who care for him, particularly on admission to a specialist unit – but anything we can do to encourage the deep and loving relationship between the mother and her baby (and which can include the father too) has to be as important as the technical expertise at our fingertips. Being skilled in breastfeeding is every bit as important as being skilled in the intricacies of supporting a baby needing ventilation. Mothers will remember for the rest of their lives the first skin contact, the first time their baby searches for the breast and the first breastfeed, and the knowledge that they contributed such a vital part of their baby's recovery and continuing development.

9.1.1 Staff education

In order to help the mothers and their babies in our neonatal and other specialist units to succeed in breastfeeding, the staff who care for them have to be both skilled and knowledgeable. The following suggestions aim to make the process of education available to all members of staff, and encourage units to have a practical approach to lactation management and training.

1. A comprehensive and practical set of breastfeeding guidelines, appropriate to the needs of babies on a neonatal or paediatric unit or in any other specialist area, should be available to all staff, nursing and

medical. These guidelines should incorporate or reflect the breast-feeding policy or guidelines of the maternity unit, so that the mothers are given consistent advice by the staff of all clinical areas. The guidelines should be based on the Baby Friendly Hospital Initiative *Ten Steps* (Box 9.1). Because of the different backgrounds of the staff who work in various specialist units, it is important that the guidelines do not assume any prior knowledge of lactation.

2. A set of up-to-date reference materials (books, slides and videos) on lactation and infant feeding should be available to staff, for private study, reference and to guide the policies of a particular clinical area. The books marked with an asterisk in the appendix would be particularly useful in a neonatal or paediatric unit.

3. Regular in-service training sessions should be held which update staff and ensure that practical skills are continually assessed (in the same way as other skills relating to neonatal nursing are assessed). These could be organized between the community, maternity, paediatric and neonatal units to encourage cooperation between staff, and to provide a forum for sharing the different experiences of breastfeeding of their staff members.

Box 9.1 Ten steps to successful breastfeeding

Step 1 Have a written breastfeeding policy that is routinely communicated to all healthcare staff

Step 2 Train all healthcare staff in skills necessary to implement this policy

Step 3 Inform all pregnant women about the benefits and management of breastfeeding

Step 4 Help mothers initiate breastfeeding within half an hour of birth

Step 5 Show mothers how to breastfeed, and how to maintain lactation even if they are separated from their infants

Step 6 Give newborn infants no food or drink other than breastmilk, unless medically indicated

Step 7 Practise 'rooming-in' – allow mothers and infants to remain together 24 hours a day

Step 8 Encourage breastfeeding on demand

Step 9 Give no artificial teats or pacifiers ('dummies' or soothers) to breastfeeding infants

Step 10 Foster the establishment of breastfeeding support groups, and refer mothers to them on discharge from the hospital or clinic

4. Basic lactational management and skill training should be given in all the training and orientation programmes for new staff choosing to work in neonatal, maternity or paediatric units.

5. To ensure all neonatal and paediatric unit staff receive adequate practical training in lactation, a workbook could be used in which a number of practical skills are recorded: for example, all staff to observe at least 15 normal complete breastfeeds on a maternity unit; observe five mothers hand-expressing and five mothers using a mechanical pump; observe 15 mothers and their preterm babies in the process of establishing breastfeeding; any abnormal breast physiology observed could be recorded. A second section could be devoted to assisting mothers and their babies. This booklet could be part of the basic training requirements alongside any other similar course requirements in the speciality. Midwives, for example, already use such a book through-out their basic training to record number of antenatal examinations performed, deliveries observed and conducted, and postnatal checks undertaken.

6. Encourage members of staff to attend a specialized breastfeeding training course, such as the three-day UK Baby Friendly Initiative 'Breastfeeding Management' modular course (for more information contact UNICEF UK) or the four-week 'Breastfeeding: Practice and Policy' course held in London each July at the Centre for International Child Health, Institute of Child Health (for addresses, see appendix). This will ensure there is a pool of people with specialized knowledge on the unit who can teach their colleagues and help mothers as well.

7. Unit audits of the effectiveness of feeding policies should be undertaken at regular intervals. These may be conducted alongside other audits, which are already undertaken, and any changes to policies made if necessary. Records of mothers' feeding intentions and outcomes should be held.

8. All neonatal and paediatric unit staff should be aware of the Baby Friendly Hospital Initiative (BFHI) and ensure that the list *Ten Steps to Successful Breastfeeding* is displayed in the maternity unit (Box 9.1). These steps provide good practice guidelines and should be implemented whether or not the hospital is working towards the BFHI award. There is also a set of UK paediatric guidelines which should shape the breastfeeding practices in paediatric units and can also be used in neonatal units (Box 9.2).

9.1.2 The neonatal unit

In addition to increasing staff awareness of the important theoretical and practical aspects of lactation, the neonatal or paediatric units have

---

Box 9.2 Paediatric breastfeeding: good practice guidelines

1 Have a written breastfeeding policy that is routinely communicated to all healthcare staff and provide appropriate training in the skills necessary to implement this policy

2 Provide mothers with an environment and facilities that meet their needs for privacy, information and appropriate nutrition

3 Support mothers in their choice of feeding method, assisting in the establishment and maintenance of breastfeeding

4 Provide parents with written and verbal information about the benefits of breastfeeding and breastmilk

5 Use alternative techniques conducive to breastfeeding if a baby is unable to feed at the breast

6 Give no bottles or dummies to breastfeeding babies unless medically indicated and with parents' permission

7 Provide facilities that allow parents and babies to be together 24 hours a day in order to promote breastfeeding on demand

8 Plan all nursing and medical care to minimize disturbance to the breastfeeding relationship

9 Provide mothers with a dedicated facility that is appropriately furnished with well-maintained and sterilized equipment for the safe expression and storage of breastmilk

10 Provide parents with information about breastfeeding support groups during admission and on discharge from hospital

---

These paediatric guidelines are based on the UNICEF Baby Friendly Hospital Initiative 'Ten Steps'. They represent the work of the UK Multidisciplinary Paediatric Breastfeeding Working Party. Celia Shore, who sadly died in 1997, was the chairperson of this working party and deserves special mention for her huge contribution to these guidelines.

---

to promote a positive atmosphere towards breastfeeding. This can be achieved in the following ways:

1. On each working shift, one member of staff could be designated to be responsible for the care of lactating and breastfeeding mothers.

2. A 'no-bottle' policy should be adopted for babies to be breastfed, unless bottles are specifically requested by the parents.

3. A room should be made available for mothers who wish to express or breastfeed in private, preferably with facilities for making drinks, or

adequate screens provided for mothers who wish to express or breastfeed in private, when a specific room is not available.

4. Ensure that mothers do not have to go a long distance from the unit for meals, and risk missing a feed. Facilities where a mother can buy or eat food near or on the unit are helpful. The provision of a microwave or small kitchen would be helpful.

5. Make general information about breastfeeding and other feeding methods available to parents. This information could be put on a notice-board for parents to read at their leisure. Pamphlets from the various support groups should be readily available, such as those from the Breastfeeding Network, National Childbirth Trust, La Leche League and the Association of Breastfeeding Mothers, and also specialist leaflets, for example from the Cleft Lip and Palate Association. Posters are available from the Royal College of Midwives and the Baby Friendly Initiative, UNICEF UK. Alternatively, photographs taken on the particular unit could form the basis of the information given. Responsibility for the board could be rotated among the staff.

6. The nursing notes relating to the baby's care should contain a section documenting the advice and practical help in lactation given to a mother. This could form part of any care plan, so that it is updated on a daily basis.

7. An infant feeding specialist is recommended for the neonatal unit. Their role could incorporate the breastfeeding needs of the maternity and paediatric units. They could be a resource person for both staff and parents, and provide support and help to the community midwives, health visitors, practice nurses and general practitioners.

8. Fully implement the World Health Organization International Code of Marketing of Breastmilk Substitutes.[1] Branded milks should not be on display, and no posters from formula milk companies should be used to promote either breast feeding or bottle-feeding. No cot cards, growth charts, note pads, diary covers, pens or other material should be used carrying formula-milk company logos.

9. Alternative feeding devices, such as breastfeeding supplementers and cups, should be provided.

10. Encourage the setting up of a local milk bank. This will ensure that all babies have the opportunity of receiving breastmilk throughout their hospital stay.

It may seem idealistic to suggest that more staff should be employed, such as a feeding specialist to help mothers achieve success in breastfeeding. However, breastfeeding has to be seen in the context of long-term benefits rather than short-term gains. If, for example, fewer mothers suffer breast cancer or hip fractures, and fewer babies are admitted to paediatric units with gastrointestinalillness or otitis media, then it is an investment in the future health of the population.

9.1.3 Helping the parents

Further measures that would specifically help parents, and particularly mothers, include:

1. The provision of information booklets based on the unit breast-feeding guidelines, which give clear and simple information. This information should be available in different languages if appropriate. (Similar booklets could be available on bottle-feeding for parents wishing to feed their baby in this way, for they also need to be taught to use bottles correctly.)

2. A designated member of staff (not necessarily the person looking after the baby) should give the mother the help and advice she requires on lactation, as soon as possible after delivery. To ensure continuity, this member of staff should, where possible, provide the advice to the mother throughout her baby's stay on the unit.

3. A support group for breastfeeding mothers (and their partners) would help overcome some of the feelings of isolation these mothers can experience. This could be organized initially by the staff of a unit or by one of the voluntary breastfeeding counsellor organizations. It could gradually be given over to the parents themselves to run. It is helpful for this to take place in the hospital and for a member of staff also to attend – to offer any help or advice that may be sought.

4. Have regular group sessions on breastfeeding for mothers on the unit. Topics such as positioning, attachment and expression should be included as core subject areas. Dolls could be used for practising different positions.

5. Have regular video sessions. Show videos on cup-feeding, feeding cues and bathing with the baby to a group of mothers and encourage discussion afterwards. These sessions should take place with a member of staff present.

6. Mothers who are expressing breastmilk or breastfeeding require the support of a range of people. Breastfeeding counsellors from one of the lay breastfeeding organizations can provide continuing support and care, both while the baby is in hospital and after discharge. Therefore, the mother should be put in touch with a counsellor during the baby's stay in hospital.

7. Parents could be asked to give written permission for the use of dummies or pacifiers or bottles to be used if the baby is to be breastfed.

REFERENCE

1. Sokol EJ (1997) *The Code Handbook. A Guide to Implementing the International Code of Marketing of Breastmilk Substitutes.* Penang: International Code Documentation Centre.

Appendix
Breastfeeding support

SUPPORT GROUPS IN THE UK

Association of Breastfeeding Mothers
PO Box 207
Bridgewater TA6 7YT
Telephone 0207 813 1481
E-mail: abm@clara.net

Breastfeeding Network
PO Box 11136
Paisley PA2 8YB
Telephone 0870 900 878 (line open 0930 to 2130)

La Leche League
Breastfeeding Help and Information
PO Box BM 3424
London WC1 6XX
Telephone 0207 242 1278

National Childbirth Trust
Alexandra House
Oldham Terrace
London W3 6NH
Telephone 0870 444 8707

OTHER USEFUL ADDRESSES

Baby Milk Action Coalition
5 St Andrews Place
Cambridge CB2 3AX
Telephone 01223 464420

British Council of Complementary Therapies
PO Box 194
London SE16 1Q2
Telephone 0207 237 5165

British Homoeopathic Association
27a Devonshire Street
London W1N 1RJ
Telephone 0207 935 2163

Centre for International Child Health
Institute of Child Health
30 Guilford Street
London WC1N 1EH
http://www.cich.ich.ucl.ac.uk

Cleft Lip and Palate Association
235–237 Finchley Road
London NW3 6LS
Telephone 0207 431 0033
http://www.clapa.com (information available about breastfeeding)

Multiple Births Foundation
Queen Charlotte's and Chelsea Hospital
Goldhawk Road
London W6 0XG
Telephone 0208 383 3519
E-mail: mbf@rpms.ac.uk

Twins and Multiple Births Association (TAMBA)
PO Box 30
Little Sutton
The Wirral L66 1TH
Telephone 0151 348 0020
TAMBA Twinline 01732 868000

UNICEF UK Baby Friendly Initiative
Africa House
64–78 Kingsway
London WC2B 6NB
Telephone 0207 312 7652
E-mail: bfi@unicef.org.uk

United Kingdom Association for Milk Banking
The Milk Bank
Queen Charlotte's and Chelsea Hospital
Du Cane Road
London W12 0HS
Telephone 0208 383 3559
E-mail: ukamb@science-network.com

USEFUL LITERATURE

Akre J (ed.) (1992) *Infant Feeding – The Physiological Basis* Geneva: WHO. ISBN 92-4-068670-3

*Hale T (2000) *Medications and Mothers' Milk*. 9th edn. Amarillo: Pharmasoft Medical Publishing. ISBN 0-9636219-3-9

Helsing E, Savage-King F (1985) *Breastfeeding in Practice*. Oxford: Oxford University Press. ISBN 0-19-261485-1

Henschel D, Inch S (1996) *Breastfeeding: A Guide for Midwives*. Hale: Books for Midwives Press. ISBN 1-898507-12-0

Herzog-Isler C, Honigmann K (1996) *Give Us A Little Time*. Baar: Medela AG. ISBN 3-9521120-2-X

La Leche League (1997*) The Womanly Art of Breast Feeding,* 6th edn. Franklin: La Leche League International. ISBN 0-912500-24-7

*La Leche League International (1997) The *Breastfeeding Answer Book*. Schaumburg: La Leche League. ISBN 0-912500-48-4

*Lawrence RA, Lawrence RM (1999) *Breastfeeding: A Guide for the Medical Profession,* 5th edn. London: Mosby. ISBN 0-8151-2615-8

Lothrop H, Moody J, Britten J, Hogg K (1997) *Breastfeeding Your Baby*. National Childbirth Trust Guide. Cambridge: Fisher Books. ISBN 1-555611-22-2

Minchin M (1998) *Breastfeeding Matters,* 4th edn. St Kilda: Alma Publications. ISBN 0-9593183-3-X

Palmer G (1993) *The Politics of Breastfeeding,* 2nd edn. London: Pandora Press. ISBN 0-04-440877-3

*Renfrew M, Fisher C, Armes S (2000) *Bestfeeding. Getting Breastfeeding Right for You*, 2nd edn. Berkeley: Celestial Arts. ISBN 0-89087-955-9

Riordan J (1991) *A Practical Guide to Breastfeeding.* London: Jones & Bartlett. ISBN 0-86720-448-6

Riordan J, Auerbach K (1999) *Breastfeeding and Human Lactation*, 2nd edn. London: Jones & Bartlett. ISBN 0-763705-45-4

Royal College of Midwives (2002) *Successful Breastfeeding,* 3rd edn. Edinburgh: Churchill Livingstone. ISBN 0-443-05967-5

Smale M (1999) *The National Trust Book of Breast-feeding,* 2nd edn. London: Vermilion. ISBN 0-09-182569-5

Stanway P, Stanway A (1988) *Breast is Best.* London: Pan Books. ISBN 0330-28110-0

*United Kingdom Association for Milk Banking (2001) *Guidelines for the Collection, Storage and Handling of Breast Milk for a Mother's Own Baby on a Neonatal Unit,* 2nd edn. London: UKAMB.

*United Kingdom Association for Milk Banking (1999) *Guidelines for the Establishment and Operation of Human Milk Banks in the UK,* 2nd edn. London: UKAMB.

Vincent P (1999) *Feeding Our Babies.* Hale: Hochland & Hochland. ISBN 1-898507-64-3

WHO Working Group on Infant Growth (1994) *An Evaluation of Infant Growth.* Geneva: WHO Nutrition Unit.

*World Health Organization (1997) *Hypoglycaemia of the Newborn. Review of the Literature.* WHO/CHD/97.1. Geneva: WHO.

World Health Organization (1998) *Evidence for the Ten Steps to Successful Breastfeeding.* WHO/CHD/98.9. Geneva: WHO.

*World Health Organization (1998) *Relactation. A Review of Experience and Recommendations for Practice.* WHO/CHS/CAH/ 98.14. Geneva: WHO.

*World Health Organization (2000) *Mastitis. Causes and Management.* WHO/FCH/CAH/00.13. Geneva: WHO.

*Books recommended for reference in a neonatal or paediatric unit.

Other sources of information

Breastfeeding Abstracts. Published quarterly by La Leche League International. Obtainable from the national organization for a small annual subscription.

Breastfeeding Briefs. Published quarterly by GIFA, Box 157, 1211 Geneva 19, Switzerland.

USEFUL VIDEOS

Matt and Mandy: A solution for breastfeeding attachment through co-bathing (1994) Produced by Heather Harris, Melbourne.
Contact: http://www.acegraphics.com.au

Breast is Best (1994) Produced by the Norwegian Health Board.
(35 minutes)
Contact: http://www.acegraphics.com.au

Infant Cues – A feeding guide (1998) Mark-it TV
Contact: market.television@btinternet.com

Samuel: Breastfed infants with cleft lip and cleft palate. Available from Christa Herzog-Isler, Pilatusstrasse 4, CH-6033 Buchrain. Switzerland.
Telephone +41 440 22 14

CD-ROM

Breastfeeding: A multimedia learning resource for healthcare professionals (1998) Spencer SA, Jones E, Woods A. Matrix Multimedia: http://www.MatrixMultimedia.co.uk.

Index